Frailty

Guest Editor

JEREMY D. WALSTON, MD

CLINICS IN
GERIATRIC MEDICINE

www.geriatric.theclinics.com

February 2011 • Volume 27 • Number 1

SAUNDERS an imprint of ELSEVIER, Inc.

W.B. SAUNDERS COMPANY
A Division of Elsevier Inc.

1600 John F. Kennedy Blvd., Suite 1800. Philadelphia, Pennsylvania 19103-2899

http://www.theclinics.com

CLINICS IN GERIATRIC MEDICINE Volume 27, Number 1
February 2011 ISSN 0749–0690, ISBN-13: 978-1-4377-2452-3

Editor: Yonah Korngold
Developmental Editor: Donald E. Mumford

Clinics in Geriatric Medicine (ISSN 0749-0690) is published quarterly by Elsevier Inc., 360 Park Avenue South, New York, NY 10010-1710. Months of issue are February, May, August, and November. Business and Editorial Offices: 1600 John F. Kennedy Blvd., Suite 1800, Philadelphia, PA 191023-2899. Periodicals postage paid at New York, NY, and additional mailing offices. Subscription prices is $241.00 per year (US individuals), $427.00 per year (US institutions), $167.00 per year (US student/resident), $314.00 per year (Canadian individuals), $532.00 per year (Canadian institutions), $333.00 per year (foreign individuals) and $532.00 per year (foreign institutions). Foreign air speed delivery is included in all *Clinics* subscription prices. All prices are subject to change without notice. POSTMASTER: Send address changes to *Clinics in Geriatric Medicine*, Elsevier Health Sciences Division, Subscription Customer Service, 3251 Riverport Lane, Maryland Heights, MO 63043. Telephone: 1-800-654-2452 (U.S. and Canada); 314-447-8871 (outside U.S. and Canada). Fax: 314-447-8029. E-mail: journalscustomer service-usa@elsevier.com (for print support) or journalsonlinesupport-usa@elsevier.com (for online support).

Reprints. For copies of 100 or more, of articles in this publication, please contact the Commercial Reprints Department, Elsevier Inc., 360 Park Avenue South, New York, New York 10010-1710. Tel.: (212) 633-3812; Fax: (212) 462-1935, email: reprints@elsevier.com.

Clinics in Geriatric Medicine is covered in *MEDLINE/PubMed (Index Medicus)*, *EMBASE/Excerpta Medica*, *Current Contents/Clinical Medicine (CC/CM)*, and the *Cumulative Index to Nursing & Allied Health Literature.*

Printed in the United States of America
Transferred to Digital Printing, 2011

Contributors

GUEST EDITOR

JEREMY D. WALSTON, MD
Raymond and Anna Lublin Professor of Medicine, Division of Geriatric Medicine and Gerontology, Johns Hopkins University School of Medicine, Baltimore, Maryland

AUTHORS

PETER M. ABADIR, MD
Division of Geriatric Medicine and Gerontology, Johns Hopkins University School of Medicine, Baltimore, Maryland

NEAL S. FEDARKO, PhD
Director, Translational Research Training Program in Gerontology & Geriatrics; Co-Director, Biology of Frailty Program; Professor of Medicine, Division of Geriatric Medicine and Gerontology, Department of Medicine, Johns Hopkins University School of Medicine, Johns Hopkins University, Baltimore, Maryland

ROGER A. FIELDING, PhD
Senior Scientist and Director, Nutrition, Exercise Physiology and Sarcopenia Laboratory, Jean Mayer USDA Human Nutrition Research Center on Aging, Tufts University, Boston, Massachusetts

FRED CHAU-YANG KO, MD
Assistant Professor, Department of Geriatrics and Palliative Medicine, Mount Sinai School of Medicine, New York, New York

SEAN X. LENG, MD, PhD
Associate Professor of Medicine, Division of Geriatric Medicine and Gerontology, Department of Medicine, Johns Hopkins University School of Medicine, Baltimore, Maryland

HUIFEN LI, PhD
Research Associate, Division of Geriatric Medicine and Gerontology, Department of Medicine, Johns Hopkins University School of Medicine, Baltimore, Maryland

CHRISTINE K. LIU, MD
Fellow in Geriatrics, Section of Geriatrics, Department of Medicine, Boston University School of Medicine; Nutrition, Exercise Physiology and Sarcopenia Laboratory, Jean Mayer USDA Human Nutrition Research Center on Aging, Tufts University, Boston, Massachusetts

ARNOLD MITNITSKI, PhD
Division of Geriatric Medicine, Dalhousie University, Halifax, Nova Scotia, Canada

KENNETH ROCKWOOD, MD, FRCPC, FRCP
Professor of Medicine (Geriatric Medicine and Neurology), Kathryn Allen Weldon
Professor of Alzheimer Research, Division of Geriatric Medicine, Dalhousie University,
Halifax, Nova Scotia, Canada

CINDY N. ROY, PhD
Assistant Professor, Division of Geriatric Medicine and Gerontology, Department of
Medicine, Johns Hopkins University School of Medicine, Baltimore, Maryland

CARLOS O. WEISS, MD, MHS
Assistant Professor of Medicine, Division of Geriatric Medicine and Gerontology,
Johns Hopkins School of Medicine; Center on Aging and Health, Johns Hopkins
Medical Institutions, Baltimore, Maryland

QIAN-LI XUE, PhD
Assistant Professor of Medicine, Department of Medicine, Johns Hopkins University
School of Medicine, Baltimore, Maryland

XU YAO, MD
Postdoctoral Fellow, Divisions of Allergy & Clinical Immunology and Geriatric Medicine
and Gerontology, Johns Hopkins University School of Medicine, Baltimore, Maryland;
Associate Professor, Division of Clinical Dermatology, Institute of Dermatology and Skin
Diseases Hospital, Peking Union Medical College and Chinese Academy of Medical
Sciences, Nanjing, China

Contents

> This article reviews the current state of knowledge regarding the epidemiology of frailty by focusing on 6 specific areas: (1) clinical definitions of frailty, (2) evidence of frailty as a medical syndrome, (3) prevalence and incidence of frailty by age, gender, race, and ethnicity, (4) transitions between discrete frailty states, (5) natural history of manifestations of frailty criteria, and (6) behavior modifications as precursors to the development of clinical frailty.

> As nonreplicative cells age, they commonly accumulate subcellular deficits that can compromise function. As people age, they too experience problems that can accumulate. As deficits (symptoms, signs, illnesses, disabilities) accumulate, people become more susceptible to adverse health outcomes, including worse health and even death. This state of increased risk of adverse health outcomes is indistinguishable from the idea of frailty, so deficit accumulation represents another way to define frailty. Counting deficits not only allows grades of frailty to be discerned but also provides insights into the complex problems of older adults. This process is potentially useful to geriatricians who need to be experts in managing complexity. A key to managing complexity is through instruments such as a comprehensive geriatric assessment, which can serve as the basis for routine clinical estimation of an individual's degree of frailty. Understanding people and their needs as deficits accumulate is an exciting challenge for clinical research on frailty and its management by geriatricians.

> In developing and validating the concept of frailty as a geriatric syndrome, it has been necessary to distinguish the clinical expression of frailty from normal age-related changes and other age-related disease pathologies. A framework for excluding potentially confounding disease and a working clinical tool to diagnose frailty have been provided. The associations between frailty and other pathophysiologies has also been shown. However, investigating the underlying biologic basis for the geriatric syndrome of frailty by studying basic homeostatic pathways and mechanisms has not proceeded at the same rate. The following article provides an overview of the homeostatic pathways emphasized in research on aging and explains how this science may help to stimulate frailty research.

There are two hallmarks of aging that must be considered primary concerns when trying to improve health for older adults: frailty and chronic diseases. Some pathologic mechanisms related to diseases may help to explain frailty. This article describes known associations among frailty and chronic diseases and introduces punished inefficiency as an explanatory framework for frailty. Punished inefficiency proposes that having several physiologic impairments leads to physiologic inefficiencies. These inefficiencies may become manifest as frailty, often in the presence of disease. Therefore, frail older adults perform less external work because they must spend more on an absolute scale out of a smaller pool of internal resources. Stress imposed on frail older adults strengthens this negative feedback to activity, leading to disuse. This article discusses how people with frailty and chronic diseases may experience a malignant course and thereby intends to improve the ability to identify beneficial biologic and health care delivery strategies for older adults with, or at risk of, frailty.

Over the last few decades, the understanding of the renin-angiotensin system (RAS) has advanced dramatically. RAS is now thought to play a crucial role in physiologic and pathophysiologic mechanisms in almost every organ system and is a key regulator of hypertension, cardiovascular disease, and renal function. Angiotensin II (Ang II) promotes inflammation and the generation of reactive oxygen species and governs onset and progression of vascular senescence, which are all associated with functional and structural changes, contributing to age-related diseases. Although the vast majority of the actions of Ang II, including vascular senescence, are mediated by the Ang II type 1 receptor (AT1R), the identification, characterization, and cloning of the angiotensin type 2 receptor has focused attention on this receptor and to its antagonistic effect on the detrimental effects of AT1R. This review provides an overview of the changes in RAS with aging and age-disease interactions culminating in the development of frailty.

Although anemia is regarded as a relatively common occurrence in older adults, the vigor with which the medical community should intervene to correct this common problem is disputed. Epidemiologic data clearly correlate anemia with functional decline, disability, and mortality. Anemia may contribute to functional decline by restricting oxygen delivery to muscle, or to cognitive decline by restricting oxygen delivery to the brain. On the other hand, the erythron may be a separate target of the same biologic mediators that influence deterioration of physiologic systems that contribute to weakness, functional and cognitive decline, and mortality. Clinical trials aimed at treating anemia in older adults could assess whether physical performance is improved or whether mortality risk declines with improved hemoglobin, but sufficient evidence from such trials is currently lacking.

With few guidelines regarding treatment of older adults and significant risk for adverse events associated with transfusion and erythroid stimulating agents, anemia often goes untreated or ignored in geriatric clinics. This article reviews the problem of anemia in older adults, with a particular emphasis on the frail elderly. The gaps in the evidence base for the treatment of anemia in older adults are reviewed and the options for advancing the field are assessed.

Inflammation and Immune System Alterations in Frailty

Xu Yao, Huifen Li, and Sean X. Leng

Frailty is an important geriatric syndrome characterized by multisystem dysregulation. Substantial evidence suggests heightened inflammatory state and significant immune system alterations in frailty. A heightened inflammatory state is marked by increases in levels of inflammatory molecules (interleukin 6 and C-reactive protein) and counts of white blood cell and its subpopulations, which may play an important role in the pathogenesis of frailty, directly or through its detrimental influence on other physiologic systems. Alterations in the innate immune system include decreased proliferation of the peripheral blood mononuclear cells and upregulated monocytic expression of specific stress-responsive inflammatory pathway genes. In the adaptive immune system, although little information is available about potential B-cell changes, significant alterations have been identified in the T-cell compartment, including increased counts of CD8+, CD8+CD28–, CCR5+T cells, above and beyond age-related senescent immune remodeling.

The Clinical Care of Frail, Older Adults

Fred Chau-Yang Ko

Frailty and its management represent an emerging area of clinical care in older adults. Geriatricians have long recognized a syndrome of multiple comorbid conditions, immobility, weakness, and poor tolerance of physiologic stressors in older adults. Patients with these characteristics are described as frail and suffer increased adverse clinical outcomes. This article reviews the clinical spectrum of frailty in older adults, its biologic etiology, and potential clinical interventions. Several operational definitions of frailty and the associated clinical signs, symptoms, and outcomes are outlined. The biologic mechanisms hypothesized to underlie frailty are explored, particularly in the musculoskeletal, endocrine, and immune systems. Treatment options for frail, older adults are discussed, including physiologic system-targeted interventions and geriatric models of care.

Exercise as an Intervention for Frailty

Christine K. Liu and Roger A. Fielding

By 2015, nearly 15% of the US population will be older than 65 years. In 2030, there will be more than 70 million older Americans. This increase in the elderly population has prompted interest in recent years toward the study of frail older adults. This article reviews the literature investigating the utility of aerobic and resistance exercise training as an intervention for frailty in older adults. In addition, areas of future research are addressed, including concerns related to the dissemination of exercise interventions on a widespread scale. Guidelines for an "exercise prescription" for frail older adults are briefly outlined.

THE CLINICS ARE NOW AVAILABLE ONLINE!

Access your subscription at:
www.theclinics.com

Preface

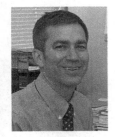

Jeremy D. Walston, MD
Guest Editor

As the population ages and more individuals are living well past age 80, maintaining a functional, independent, and high-quality life in the community will be an increasingly important goal for older adults and for society in general. Frailty is a syndrome of late-life decline and vulnerability that serves as a warning sign for adverse health outcomes and for mortality. The identification of vulnerable, frail, adults may allow for the development of preventive interventions that help to maintain good health and high quality of life well into the 8th and 9th decade of life. Over the past several years, investigators from across the country have been attempting to better define frailty through describing its clinical and biological characteristics. A number of clinical screening tools have been developed that help to identify the most vulnerable older adults, and inflammatory, muscle, and neuroendocrine dysregulation has been described as characteristic of frailty. In this edition of *Clinical Geriatric Medicine*, the authors have provided rich summaries of current models and definitions of frailty, of how age and chronic disease impact the development of frailty, and of how inflammation, anemia, the renin-angiotensin system, and immune system changes may impact or mark frailty. The final articles discuss potential clinical interventions that may benefit frail, older adults, including focused health care models and exercise interventions that may attenuate vulnerability. The articles in this issue were developed to help clinicians and investigators better understand the progress that has been made in this field, and to foster a broader research effort focused on the prevention and treatment of frailty.

Jeremy D. Walston, MD
Division of Geriatric Medicine and Gerontology
Johns Hopkins University School of Medicine
John R. Burton Pavilion
5505 Hopkins Bayview Circle
Baltimore, MD 21224, USA

E-mail address:
jwalston@jhmi.edu

Clin Geriatr Med 27 (2011) xi
doi:10.1016/j.cger.2010.09.001
0749-0690/11/$ — see front matter © 2011 Elsevier Inc. All rights reserved.

geriatric.theclinics.com

The Frailty Syndrome: Definition and Natural History

Qian-Li Xue, PhD

KEYWORDS

- Clinical phenotype • Hazard ratio • Frailty
- Latent class analysis

Frailty is a common clinical syndrome in older adults, which carries an increased risk for poor health outcomes, including falls, incident disability, hospitalization, and mortality.[1–5] Elucidating its cause and natural history is therefore critical for identifying high-risk subsets and new arenas for frailty prevention and treatment.

In an attempt to standardize and operationalize the definition of frailty, Fried and colleagues[2] proposed a clinical phenotype of frailty as a well-defined syndrome with biologic underpinnings. These investigators hypothesized that the clinical manifestations of frailty are related in a mutually exacerbating cycle of negative energy balance, sarcopenia, and diminished strength and tolerance for exertion. Building on this conceptual framework, preliminary evidence has now been obtained on the natural history of the clinical phenotype of frailty.[3,6] This article reviews the current state of knowledge regarding the epidemiology of frailty by focusing on 6 specific areas: (1) clinical definitions of frailty, (2) evidence of frailty as a medical syndrome, (3) prevalence and incidence of frailty by age, gender, race, and ethnicity, (4) transitions between discrete frailty states, (5) natural history of manifestations of frailty criteria, and (6) behavior modifications as precursors to the development of clinical frailty.

DEFINITION OF FRAILTY

Frailty is theoretically defined as a clinically recognizable state of increased vulnerability, resulting from aging-associated decline in reserve and function across multiple physiologic systems such that the ability to cope with everyday or acute stressors is compromised. In the absence of a gold standard, frailty has been operationally defined by Fried and colleagues[2] as a condition meeting 3 of the 5 phenotypic criteria indicating compromised energetics, namely, low grip strength, low energy, slowed waking speed, low physical activity, and unintentional weight loss (**Table 1**). A prefrail stage, in which 1 or 2 criteria are present, identifies a subset at high risk of progressing to frailty. Various adaptations of the clinical phenotype described by Fried have

Department of Medicine, Johns Hopkins University School of Medicine, 2024 East Monument Street, Suite 2-700, Baltimore, MD 21205-1179, USA
E-mail address: qxue@jhsph.edu

Table 1

Comparison of the frailty-defining criteria defined by the Cardiovascular Health Study and the Women's Health and Aging Studies

Characteristics	Cardiovascular Health Study	Women's Health and Aging Studies
Weight loss	Baseline: lost >4.5 kg unintentionally in the last year Follow-up: ([weight in previous year − current weight]/[weight in previous year])≥0.05 and the loss was unintentional	Baseline: either of the following: ([weight at age 60 y − weight at examination]/[weight at age 60 years])≥0.1 BMI at examination<18.5 Follow-up: either of the following: BMI at examination<18.5 ([weight in previous year − current weight]/[weight in previous year])≥0.05 and the loss was unintentional
Exhaustion	Self-report of either Feeling that everything the person did was an effort in the last week Inability to get going in the last week	Self-report of any of the following: Low usual energy level[a] (≤3, range 0–10) Felt unusually tired in the past month[b] Felt unusually weak in the past month[b]
Low physical activity	Women: energy<270 kcal on activity scale (18 items) Men: energy<383 kcal on activity scale (18 items)	Women: energy<90 kcal on activity scale (6 items) Men: energy<128 kcal on activity scale (6 items)
Slowness	Observed when walking 4.57 m at usual pace Women Time≥7 s for height≤159 cm Time≥6 s for height>159 cm Men Time≥7 s for height≤173 cm Time≥6 s for height>173 cm	Observed when walking 4 m at usual pace Women Speed≤4.57/7 m/s for height≤159 cm Speed≤4.57/6 m/s for height>159 cm Men Speed≤4.57/7 m/s for height≤173 cm Speed≤4.57/6 m/s for height>173 cm

Weakness	Grip strength	Grip strength: same as in CHS
	Women	
	≤ 17 kg for BMI ≤ 23	
	≤ 17.3 kg for BMI 23.1–26	
	≤ 18 kg for BMI 26.1–29	
	≤ 21 kg for BMI>29	
	Men	
	≤ 29 kg for BMI ≤ 24	
	≤ 30 kg for BMI 24.1–26	
	≤ 30 kg for BMI 26.1–28	
	≤ 32 kg for BMI>28	

BMI: Body mass index; calculated as the weight in kilograms divided by the height in meters squared.

[a] Rated on 0–10 scale, where 0 indicated "no energy" and 10 indicated "the most energy that you have ever had."

[b] If yes, there followed the question, "How much of the time?" the feeling persisted; responses "Most" or "All" of the time were considered indicative of exhaustion.

emerged in the literature, which were often motivated by available measures in specific studies rather than meaningful conceptual differences.

Alternatively, frailty has been operationalized as a risk index by counting the number of deficits accumulated over time, termed frailty index (FI), including disability, diseases, physical and cognitive impairments, psychosocial risk factors, and geriatric syndromes (eg, falls, delirium, and urinary incontinence).[7] Compared with the Fried frailty phenotype, the FI is a more sensitive predictor of adverse health outcomes because of its finer graded risk scale and its robustness in clinical inferences with regard to the number and actual composition of the items in it.[8]

However, the discussion of the epidemiology of frailty in this article focuses on the Fried definition of frailty phenotype for several reasons. First, there is increasing consensus that frailty is a definable clinical state involving multiple signs and symptoms. Second, the clinical manifestations of frailty, in theory, may be organized into a self-perpetuating cycle of naturally progressing events (**Fig. 1**) consistent with clinical observations.[2,9] Third, converging lines of evidence suggest that these manifestations exhibit associations[10–15] that are consistent with a syndromal presentation.[1] Fourth, all the 3 reasons mentioned earlier provides a priori theoretical framework that facilitates the investigation of mechanisms underlying the development of frailty.[16] Last, it could be argued that the 5-component phenotype is more appealing for use in a clinical setting than the FI that typically contains 30 to 70 items.

NATURAL HISTORY OF MANIFESTATIONS OF FRAILTY CRITERIA

Understanding the points of onset of frailty is vital to early identification of at-risk individuals and intervention on those components that are first affected, when reversal

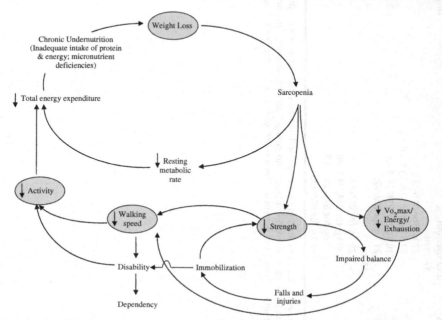

Fig. 1. Cycle of frailty. (Xue QL, Bandeen-Roche K, Varadhan R, et al. Initial manifestations of frailty criteria and the development of frailty phenotype in the Women's Health and Aging Study II. J Gerontol A Biol Sci Med Sci 2008;63(9):984–90, by permission of the Gerontological Society of America.)

may be most possible. Preclinical detection of early manifestations leading to the frailty syndrome requires an understanding of the natural history of frailty development. The author suggests 2 potential hypotheses as to the natural history of frailty initiation and progression. The author hypothesized that the cycle of frailty could be initiated via any of the clinical manifestations, which could then precipitate a vicious cycle culminating in an aggregate syndrome; and different initial manifestations may lead to differential rates of progression to frailty. Based on a 7.5-year longitudinal study of 420 participants of the Women's Health and Aging Studies (WHAS) II who were defined as nonfrail using the Fried definition of frailty phenotype at baseline, the author found initial evidence of a partially hierarchical order in the onset of frailty manifestations over time.[6] Although there was notable heterogeneity in the initial manifestations of frailty, weakness was the most common first manifestation, and occurrence of weakness, slowness, and low physical activity preceded exhaustion and weight loss in 76% of the women who were nonfrail at baseline.

The fact that weakness should presage frailty onset is consistent with earlier reports that suggest that loss of muscle strength begins in midlife.[17–19] The decline in muscle strength has been attributed to the loss of muscle mass and muscle quality, which is referred to as sarcopenia, resulting from anatomic and biochemical changes in the aging muscle.[20] The causal mechanisms underlying sarcopenia are many, including oxidative stress, dysregulation of inflammatory cytokines and hormones, malnutrition, physical inactivity, and muscle apoptosis,[21,22] all of which have been hypothesized to contribute to frailty through interactive pathways at multiple temporal and spatial scales.[16]

The finding of heterogeneity in initial criteria is consistent with the hypothesis that the cycle of frailty may be initiated by insults at many points in a hypothesized cycle of dysregulated energetics.[2,9] It was not the number of early manifestations (ie, 1 or 2) but the specific manifestations initially present that distinguished the risk and rate of onset of frailty. Specifically, women with exhaustion or weight loss as initial presenting symptoms were 3 to 5 times more likely to become frail than were women without any criterion, after adjusting for baseline age, race, education, and comorbidity. Weakness was moderately predictive of frailty onset (hazard ratio = 2.6). Neither slow walking speed nor low activity at baseline was significantly associated with incident frailty. It remains to be determined whether the different patterns of initial accumulation of frailty criteria represent different causative pathways with different rates of progression to frailty, either organ-specific or representing systemic physiologic dysregulations of aging. Alternatively, certain criterion measures may be more sensitive than others to changes associated with normal aging, for instance, performance-based criteria as opposed to self-reported criteria.

Despite heterogeneous entry points into the cycle of frailty, 80% of transitions to frailty involved adding exhaustion and/or weight loss. This finding raises the possibility that decreased energy production or increased use, as in wasting conditions, may be involved in the threshold transition in a final common pathway toward frailty. Weight loss and exhaustion rarely developed alone, but rather co-occurred with other manifestations. This co-occurrence is consistent with the reliability theory,[23] whereby an emergent aggregation of multiple frailty manifestations result from the depletion of system redundancy or compensatory mechanisms, such that any new deficit leads to the failure of the whole organism.[24–27] Then, early detection of subclinical changes or deficits at the molecular, cellular, and/or physiologic level is key to preventing or delaying the development of frailty.

The clinical utility of these findings lies in the fact that weakness was the most common initial manifestation of the frailty phenotype. It evidenced only moderate predictive validity for incident frailty. However, according to the author's conceptualization, the development of frailty is progressive and multisystemic and any 1 specific criterion alone, especially at an early stage in the process as in the case of weakness, may be neither sufficient nor specific for frailty prediction. Given that the criteria defining thresholds for grip strength are known to be associated with a greater risk of adverse outcomes, including disability and mortality,[28] weakness may nevertheless be a clinically meaningful indicator of increasing vulnerability at a relatively early stage of the frailty process, when preventive intervention could be easiest to implement and theoretically most effective. Although the subsequent or concurrent onset of weight loss or exhaustion with the other criteria may better predict frailty onset, by the time someone experiences weight loss or exhaustion, it may be too late to implement frailty interventions. Therefore, consideration should be given to the possible trade-off between risk prediction and potential for benefits in deciding the proper timing and targets of interventions.

EVIDENCE OF FRAILTY AS A MEDICAL SYNDROME

A medical syndrome is "a group of signs and symptoms that occur together and characterize a particular abnormality." To formally evaluate the degree to which the frailty phenotype conforms to the definition of a medical syndrome, Bandeen-Roche and colleagues[1] analyzed patterns of co-occurrence of the 5 frailty-defining criteria based on data from a combined sample of women aged 70 to 79 years from the WHAS I and WHAS II. Patterns of criteria co-occurrence that would support the syndrome definition are "(1) manifestation in a critical mass and (2) aggregation in a hierarchical order, as would occur in a cycle in which dysregulation in a sentinel system may trigger a cascade of alterations across other systems."[1] Propensity for criteria to co-occur in distinct subgroups would suggest the effects of distinct biologic processes rather than a syndrome. Using latent class analysis,[29] 3 population subsets (also termed classes) with similar profiles of frailty criteria co-occurrence were identified; each criterion's prevalence increased progressively across the population subsets, indicating increase in frailty severity. These findings supported the internal validity of the frailty criteria vis-à-vis the stated theory characterizing frailty as a medical syndrome and provided justification to the current counting strategy for defining frailty categories (ie, nonfrail, prefrail, and frail).

PREVALENCE AND INCIDENCE OF FRAILTY

Based on the frailty criteria developed in the Cardiovascular Health Study (CHS), the overall prevalence of frailty in community-dwelling older adults aged 65 years or older in the United States ranges from 7% to 12%. In the CHS, prevalence of frailty increased with age from 3.9% in the age group of 65 to 74 years to 25% in the age group older than 85 years and was greater in women than in men (8% vs 5%).[2] African Americans were more than twice as likely to be frail than Whites in the CHS (13% vs 6%) and the WHAS (16% vs 10%). The 1996 estimate for Mexican Americans from the Hispanic Established Populations for Epidemiologic Studies of the Elderly was 7.8%, similar to those of Whites.[4]

Similar age trends and gender differences have been reported for older adult populations in European and Latin American countries (**Table 2**). A recent survey of 7510 community-dwelling older adults in 10 European countries found that the prevalence of frailty ranged from 5.8% in Switzerland to 27% in Spain, with an overall prevalence of 17% and was higher in southern than in northern Europe, consistent with an unexplained north-south health risk gradient previously reported in the same population.[30,31]

The geographic variation in frailty prevalence among these European countries persisted after adjusting for age and gender, which led the investigators to speculate that there may be differences in cultural characteristics, influencing the perception of health and/or interpretation of the frailty questions.[30] According to a survey of 7334 older adults who were 60 years or older living in 5 large Latin American and Caribbean cities, including Bridgetown, Barbados (n = 1446); Sao Paulo, Brazil (n = 1879); Santiago, Chile (n = 1220); Havana, Cuba (n = 1726); and Mexico City, Mexico (n =1063), prevalence of frailty varied from 30% to 48% in women and from 21% to 35% in men, which was much higher than their American and European counterparts.[32]

FRAILTY TRANSITIONS

Epidemiologic data on transitions between frailty states (ie, nonfrail, prefrail, frail) were first reported by Gill and colleagues[3] in a 4.5-year longitudinal study of 754 community-living older adults who were 70 years or older. Of the 754 participants, 58% had at least 1 transition between any 2 of the 3 frailty states at one of the 3 follow-up visits 18-months apart during the study; 37%, 22%, and 9% of the participants had 1, 2, and 3 transitions. About one-third (35%) of all 18-month transitions were from states of greater frailty to states of less frailty (calculated based on data in **Table 3** of Gill and colleagues[3]). However, the likelihood of transitioning from being frail to nonfrail was extremely rare during each of the 18-month intervals.

In WHAS II, frailty status of 405 women representing two-thirds of least-disabled community-dwelling women aged 70 to 79 years was repeatedly assessed at baseline and at least one of the 4 follow-up visits spanning 7.5 years (approximately 18 months apart except for the interval between the third and the fourth examination, which was, on average, 3 years). Of the 405 women, 72% had at least 1 transition between frailty states over 7.5 years; 37%, 24%, 16%, and 2% had 1, 2, 3, and 4 transitions. Consistent with the finding of Gill and colleagues,[3] most of the transitions occurred between adjacent frailty status; one-third (34%) of all 18-month transitions were from states of greater frailty to states of less frailty. In WHAS II, the rate of transition from frail to nonfrail was noticeably higher (17%) during the first 18 months than that of the previous study, which could be because of the small sample size of the frailty group (see **Table 3**). It was also found that two-thirds of the 24 (n = 15) women who were nonfrail at baseline and became frail during the course of the study did so slowly and progressively, whereas one-third (n = 9) had rapid onset of frailty without progressing through any identified prefrail stage. This observation suggests that the rate at which frailty progresses may vary dramatically among older adults, that is, more sudden and catastrophic in some people and slowly progressive among others. Similar findings have been reported by Gill and colleagues[3] and for severe mobility disability, with the rate of progression depending on the level of comorbidity as well as specific disease types.[33] Owing to low frailty incidence, the author had limited power in detecting factors differentiating the pace of frailty development.

Because some misconstrue frailty as a premorbid state defining the end of life, the findings reported earlier suggest that frailty is not an irreversible process, certainly not an inevitable trajectory to death. Therefore, the development and evaluation of interventions designed to prevent or ameliorate frailty should remain as one of the top priorities in frailty research.

BEHAVIORAL PRECURSORS TO THE DEVELOPMENT OF FRAILTY

An overt state of frailty is believed to be preceded by behavioral adaptation made in response to declining physiologic reserve and capacity with which to meet

Table 2
Frailty prevalence and criteria in various countries

Source	Country	Number of Patients	Frailty Prevalence		Fraility Criteria
Fried et al,[2] 2001	United States	5317	Age		CHS criteria (see Table 1)
			65–74 y	3.9%	
			75–84 y	11.6%	
			Older than 85 y	25.0%	
			Sex		
			Women	8.2%	
			Men	5.2%	
			Race		
			White	5.9%	
			African American	12.9%	
Bandeen-Roche et al,[1] 2006	United States	786	Age		WHAS criteria (see Table 1)
			70–79 y	11.3%	
			Race		
			White	9.8%	
			African American	15.8%	
Santos-Eggimann et al,[30] 2009	10 European countries:	7510	Older than 65 y	17.0%	Three or more of the following 5 criteria:
	Sweden			8.6%	*Weight loss:* self-report of a diminution in the desire for food in response to the question, "What has your appetite been like?"
	Denmark			12.4%	*Exhaustion:* responding "Yes" to the question, "In the last month, have you had too little energy to do things you wanted to do?"
	Netherlands			11.3%	*Weakness:* same as in CHS
	Germany			12.1%	*Slowness:* self-report of having either "Difficulty (expected to last more than 3 months) walking 100 m" or "Climbing one flight of stairs without resting" because of health reasons
	Austria			10.8%	*Low activity:* responding "1 to 3 times a month" or "Hardly ever or never" to the question, "How often do you engage in activities that require a low or moderate level of energy, such as
	Switzerland			5.8%	
	France			15.0%	
	Italy			23.0%	
	Spain			27.3%	
	Greece			14.7%	

Graham et al,[4] 2009	United States	1996	Older than 65 y Race Mexican American	7.8%	Three or more of the following 5 criteria: *Weight loss:* unintentional weight loss of ≥4.5 kg in the last year *Exhaustion:* same as in CHS *Weakness* by grip strength: Weakest 20% for men: ≤21 kg for BMI≤24.2 ≤24.5 kg for BMI 24.3–26.8 ≤25.4 kg for BMI 26.9–29.5 ≤25.5 kg for BMI>29.5 Weakest 20% for women: ≤13.5 kg for BMI≤24.7 ≤14.2 kg for BMI 24.8–28.3 ≤15.0 kg for BMI 28.4–32.1 ≤15.0 kg for BMI>32.1 *Slowness* by 4.9-m–timed walk at fast pace Slowest 20% for men: ≥11.2 s for height ≤168 cm ≥9.7 s for height >168 cm Slowest 20% for women: ≥12.0 s for height ≤154 cm ≥11.2 s for height >154 cm *Low activity:* lowest 20th percentile on the basis of gender on the Physical Activity Scale for the Elderly Lowest 20% for men: ≤30[47] Lowest 20% for women: ≤27.5[47]

(continued on next page)

Table 2
(continued)

Source	Country	Number of Patients	Frailty Prevalence		Frailty Criteria
Alvarado et al,[32] 2008			Older than 60 y		Three or more of the following 5 criteria:
	Barbados	1446	Women	30.0%	*Weight loss:* self-report of loss of >4.5 kg unintentionally during the previous 3 months
			Men	21.5%	*Exhaustion:* responding "No" to the question, "Do you have lots of energy?" and/or responding "Yes" to the question, "Have your dropped many of your activities or interests?"
	Cuba	1726	Women	46.7%	*Weakness:* same as in CHS
			Men	26.2%	*Slowness:* self-report of difficulty in walking 100 yd and/or in climbing one flight of stairs
	Mexico	1063	Women	45.5%	*Low activity:* responding, "No" to the question, "In the last 12 mo, have your exercised regularly or participated in vigorous physical activity, such as playing a sport, dancing, or doing heavy housework, 3 or more times a week?"
			Men	30.4%	
	Chile	1220	Women	48.2%	
			Men	31.7%	
	Brazil	1879	Women	44.1%	
			Men	35.4%	
Avila-Funes et al,[44] 2009	France	6030	Older than 65 y	7.0%	Three or more of the following 5 criteria:
					Weight loss: self-report of recent loss of ≥3 kg unintentionally or BMI <21 kg/m²
					Exhaustion: same as in CHS
					Weakness: responding "Yes" to the question, "Do you have difficulty rising from a chair?"
					Slowness: gender- and height-adjusted lowest quantile on a timed 6-m walking test at usual pace
					Low activity: denied doing daily leisure activities, such as walking or gardening or participating in athletic activity at least once a week

BMI: Body mass index; calculated as the weight in kilograms divided by the height in meters squared.

Table 3
Numbers and rates of transitions according to follow-up interval

Transition	Number Baseline to 18 mo	Rate (%)	Number 18–36 mo	Rate (%)	Number 36–72 mo	Rate (%)	Number 72–90 mo	Rate (%)
Nonfrail to	N = 244		N = 222		N = 147		N = 129	
Nonfrail	179	73.4	132	59.5	93	63.3	66	51.2
Prefrail	61	25.0	86	38.7	40	27.2	58	45.0
Frail	3	1.2	4	1.8	6	4.1	2	1.6
Death	1	0.4	0	0	8	5.4	3	2.3
Prefrail to	N = 137		N = 130		N = 161		N = 130	
Nonfrail	48	35.0	26	20.0	36	22.4	22	16.9
Prefrail	75	54.7	89	68.5	92	57.1	85	65.4
Frail	9	6.6	11	8.5	15	9.3	15	11.5
Death	5	3.7	4	3.1	18	11.2	8	6.2
Frail to	N = 12		N = 13		N = 14		N = 28	
Nonfrail	2	16.7	1	0.8	2	14.3	0	0
Prefrail	7	58.3	10	76.9	5	35.7	10	35.7
Frail	2	16.7	2	15.4	7	50.0	13	46.4
Death	1	8.3	0	0	0	0	5	17.9

environmental challenges. The causes of this loss of physiologic reserve are likely to be multifactorial, including both environmental challenges (eg, area deprivation) and intraindividual challenges (eg, age-related physiologic changes). Observations of early behavioral changes during this preclinical phase in older adults in whom frailty is developing, but as yet undetected, could provide insight into the frailty development process and suggest means for early intervention. More importantly, such changes may not be captured by conventional measures of function such as fixed-distance or fixed-time walking tests for mobility function, which assess one's functional capacity under hypothetical or experimental conditions rather than enacted function in the real world.[34] Therefore, assessment of the changes in real life may reflect the net impact of declining reserve, taking into account the balance between internal physiologic capacity and external challenges older adults experience in daily life.

One example of such a behavioral precursor is life space, a measure of spatial mobility, defined as the size of the spatial area people purposely move through in their daily life as well as the frequency of travel within a specific time frame.[35,36] The author analyzed the 3-year cumulative incidence of frailty using the WHAS phenotype in relation to baseline life-space constriction among 599 community-dwelling women who were 65 years or older and not frail at baseline. Frailty-free mortality (ie, death before the observation of frailty) was treated as a competing risk. Multivariate survival models showed that when compared with women who left the neighborhood 4 or more times per week, those who left the neighborhood less frequently were 1.7 times (95% confidence interval [CI], 1.1–2.4; $P<.05$) more likely to become frail, and those who never left their homes experienced a 3-fold increase in frailty-free mortality (95% CI, 1.4–7.7; $P<.01$), after adjustment for chronic disease, physical disability, and psychosocial factors.[37] It is particularly intriguing to find that difficulty with mobility, instrumental activities of daily living, and activities of daily living alone did not necessarily lead to a reduction in life space. In fact, 97% of the participants in the study cohort had already reported mobility disability at baseline. Such discordance between functional capacity and actual performance has been reported in several other studies.[34,38,39] To explain the discrepancy, one could argue that some people may compensate for underlying functional decrements by adapting to a modified daily routine (eg, the use of assistive devices) to maintain the same level of performance in real life (ie, enacted function).[40] Although the exact reasons for this discrepancy remain unknown, the author hypothesizes that the employment of external (eg, social support) and internal (eg, using a cane) compensatory strategies (termed environmental supports and intraindividual supports, respectively, in **Fig. 2**) may help to minimize the impact of the loss of physiologic reserve and thereby preserve life-space mobility. On the other hand, the ability to compensate effectively for functional limitations may itself be a function of physiologic reserve. It may be the interplay of functional limitations and functional reserve, which determines actual function and behavior.

Obtaining empirical evidence of this association is the critical first step toward evaluating a broad conceptual framework about the cause of frailty (see **Fig. 2**). In the case of life space, it is theorized that constriction of life space is a marker of declines in physiologic reserve and that constriction of life space itself could lead to decreased physical activity and social engagement, accelerated deconditioning, and exacerbated decline in physiologic reserve, directly contributing, as these processes progress, to the development of clinical frailty and subsequent mortality. Future development of tools for the assessment of physiologic reserve and analysis of their relations to behavioral maladaptations could help in delineating the hypothesized causal pathway.

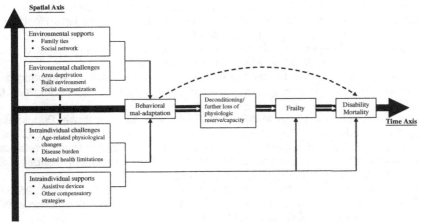

Fig. 2. Theoretical model of the association of life space with the clinical syndrome of frailty. Solid and dashed lines represent direct and indirect effects, respectively; arrows represent causal direction. (Xue QL, Fried LP, Glass TA, et al. Life-space constriction, development of frailty, and the competing risk of mortality: the Women's Health And Aging Study I. Am J Epidemiol 2008;167(2):240–8, by permission of Oxford University Press.)

SUMMARY

The recent work on the natural history of frailty has advanced the understanding of the aging process and its potential physiologic correlates. The ongoing debate on the operational definition of frailty, its subdomains (eg, physical vs cognitive), and its relationship with aging, disability, and chronic diseases[41–45] signals that more work is necessary to better define and quantify reserve and resilience, the hallmarks of frailty.[16,46] Despite this debate, researchers and clinicians have no disagreement on the severe impact of frailty on older adults, their caregivers, and on society as a whole. Although specific treatments for frailty are yet to be developed and tested, the existing clinical measures of frailty provide useful means for identifying high-risk individuals and, therefore, could lead to improved treatment, decision making, and management of care by taking into account individual vulnerabilities and propensity for adverse health outcomes.

REFERENCES

1. Bandeen-Roche K, Xue QL, Ferrucci L, et al. Phenotype of frailty: characterization in the women's health and aging studies. J Gerontol A Biol Sci Med Sci 2006; 61(3):262–6.
2. Fried LP, Tangen CM, Walston J, et al. Frailty in older adults: evidence for a phenotype. J Gerontol A Biol Sci Med Sci 2001;56(3):M146–56.
3. Gill TM, Gahbauer EA, Allore HG, et al. Transitions between frailty states among community-living older persons. Arch Intern Med 2006;166(4):418–23.
4. Graham JE, Snih SA, Berges IM, et al. Frailty and 10-year mortality in community-living Mexican American older adults. Gerontology 2009;55(6):644–51.
5. Ensrud KE, Ewing SK, Cawthon PM, et al. A comparison of frailty indexes for the prediction of falls, disability, fractures, and mortality in older men. J Am Geriatr Soc 2009;57(3):492–8.

6. Xue QL, Bandeen-Roche K, Varadhan R, et al. Initial manifestations of frailty criteria and the development of frailty phenotype in the Women's Health and Aging Study II. J Gerontol A Biol Sci Med Sci 2008;63(9):984–90.
7. Mitnitski AB, Mogilner AJ, Rockwood K. Accumulation of deficits as a proxy measure of aging. Scientific World Journal 2001;1:323–36.
8. Rockwood K, Andrew M, Mitnitski A. A comparison of two approaches to measuring frailty in elderly people. J Gerontol A Biol Sci Med Sci 2007;62:738–43.
9. Fried LP, Walston J, Hazzard WR, et al. Frailty and failure to thrive. Principles of geriatric medicine and gerontology. New York: McGraw Hill; 1998. p. 1387–402.
10. Tseng BS, Marsh DR, Hamilton MT, et al. Strength and aerobic training attenuate muscle wasting and improve resistance to the development of disability with aging. J Gerontol A Biol Sci Med Sci 1995;50:113–9.
11. Evans WJ. Exercise, nutrition, and aging. Clin Geriatr Med 1995;11(4):725–34.
12. Fleg JL, Lakatta EG. Role of muscle loss in the age-associated reduction in VO2 max. J Appl Physiol 1988;65(3):1147–51.
13. Buchner DM, Larson EB, Wagner EH, et al. Evidence for a non-linear relationship between leg strength and gait speed. Age Ageing 1996;25(5):386–91.
14. Leibel RL. Changes in energy expenditure resulting from altered body-weight. N Engl J Med 1995;332(6):621–8.
15. Morley JE. Anorexia of aging: physiologic and pathologic. Am J Clin Nutr 1997;66(4):760–73.
16. Fried LP, Hadley EC, Walston J, et al. From bedside to bench: research agenda for frailty. Sci Aging Knowledge Environ 2005;2005(31):24.
17. Nair KS. Muscle protein-turnover: methodological issues and the effect of aging. J Gerontol A Biol Sci Med Sci 1995;50:107–12.
18. Viitasalo JT, Era P, Leskinen AL, et al. Muscular strength profiles and anthropometry in random samples of men aged 31–35, 51–55 and 71–75 years. Ergonomics 1985;28(11):1563–74.
19. Lindle RS, Metter EJ, Lynch NA, et al. Age and gender comparisons of muscle strength in 654 women and men aged 20–93 yr. J Appl Physiol 1997;83(5):1581–7.
20. Kamel HK. Sarcopenia and aging. Nutr Rev 2003;61(5):157–67.
21. Marcell TJ. Sarcopenia: causes, consequences, and preventions. J Gerontol A Biol Sci Med Sci 2003;58(10):911–6.
22. Dirks AJ, Hofer T, Marzetti E, et al. Mitochondrial DNA mutations, energy metabolism and apoptosis in aging muscle. Ageing Res Rev 2006;5(2):179–95.
23. Lloyd DK, Lipow M. Reliability: management, methods, and mathematics. Englewood Cliffs (NJ): Prentice-Hall, Inc; 1962.
24. Gavrilov LA, Gavrilova NS. The reliability theory of aging and longevity. J Theor Biol 2001;213(4):527–45.
25. Bortz WM. A conceptual framework of frailty: a review. J Gerontol A Biol Sci Med Sci 2002;57(5):M283–8.
26. Amaral LA, Diaz-Guilera A, Moreira AA, et al. Emergence of complex dynamics in a simple model of signaling networks. Proc Natl Acad Sci U S A 2004;101(44):15551–5.
27. Kitano H. Systems biology: a brief overview. Science 2002;295(5560):1662–4.
28. Rantanen T, Volpato S, Ferrucci L, et al. Handgrip strength and cause-specific and total mortality in older disabled women: exploring the mechanism. J Am Geriatr Soc 2003;51(5):636–41.

29. Goodman LA. Exploratory latent structure analysis using both identifiable and unidentifiable models. Biometrika 1974;61(2):215–31.
30. Santos-Eggimann B, Cuenoud P, Spagnoli J, et al. Prevalence of frailty in middle-aged and older community-dwelling Europeans living in 10 countries. J Gerontol A Biol Sci Med Sci 2009;64(6):675–81.
31. Borsch-Supan A, Brugiavini A, Jurges H, et al. First results from the survey of health, ageing and retirement in Europe. Mannheim (Germany): Mannheim Research Institute for the Economics of Aging 8–27; 2005.
32. Alvarado BE, Zunzunegui MV, Beland F. Life course social and health conditions linked to frailty in Latin American older men and women. J Gerontol A Biol Sci Med Sci 2008;63:1399–406.
33. Guralnik JM, Ferrucci L, Balfour JL, et al. Progressive versus catastrophic loss of the ability to walk: implications for the prevention of mobility loss. J Am Geriatr Soc 2001;49(11):1463–70.
34. Glass TA. Conjugating the "tenses" of function: discordance among hypothetical, experimental, and enacted function in older adults. Gerontologist 1998;38(1): 101–12.
35. Baker PS, Bodner EV, Allman RM. Measuring life-space mobility in community-dwelling older adults. J Am Geriatr Soc 2003;51(11):1610–4.
36. May D, Nayak US, Isaacs B. The life-space diary: a measure of mobility in old people at home. Int Rehabil Med 1985;7(4):182–6.
37. Xue QL, Fried LP, Glass TA, et al. Life-space constriction, development of frailty, and the competing risk of mortality: the Women's Health and Aging Study I. Am J Epidemiol 2008;167(2):240–8.
38. Jette AM. How measurement techniques influence estimates of disability in older populations. Soc Sci Med 1994;38(7):937–42.
39. Cambois E, Robine JM, Romieu I. The influence of functional limitations and various demographic factors on self-reported activity restriction at older ages. Disabil Rehabil 2005;27(15):871–83.
40. Fried LP, Bandeen-Roche K, Chaves PHM, et al. Preclinical mobility disability predicts incident mobility disability in older women. J Gerontol A Biol Sci Med Sci 2000;55(1):M43–52.
41. Fried LP, Ferrucci L, Darer J, et al. Untangling the concepts of disability, frailty, and comorbidity: implications for improved targeting and care. J Gerontol 2004;59(3):255–63.
42. Hogan DB, MacKnight C, Bergman H. Models, definitions, and criteria of frailty. Aging Clin Exp Res 2003;15(Suppl 3):1–29.
43. Bergman H, Ferrucci L, Guralnik J, et al. Frailty: an emerging research and clinical paradigm–issues and controversies. J Gerontol 2007;62(7):731–7.
44. Avila-Funes JA, Amieva H, Barberger-Gateau P, et al. Cognitive impairment improves the predictive validity of the phenotype of frailty for adverse health outcomes: the three-city study. J Am Geriatr Soc 2009;57(3):453–61.
45. Sarkisian CA, Gruenewald TL, John Boscardin W, et al. Preliminary evidence for subdimensions of geriatric frailty: the MacArthur study of successful aging. J Am Geriatr Soc 2008;56(12):2292–7.
46. Varadhan R, Seplaki CL, Xue QL, et al. Stimulus-response paradigm for characterizing the loss of resilience in homeostatic regulation associated with frailty. Mech Ageing Dev 2008;129(11):666–70.
47. Washburn RA, Smith KW, Jette AM, et al. The Physical Activity Scale for the Elderly (PASE): development and evaluation. J Clin Epidemiol 1993;46:53–162.

Frailty Defined by Deficit Accumulation and Geriatric Medicine Defined by Frailty

Kenneth Rockwood, MD, FRCPC, FRCP*, Arnold Mitnitski, PhD

KEYWORDS

- Health deficits • Frailty • Disease presentation • Frailty index
- Comprehensive geriatric assessment • Complexity

As cells age, they develop deficits as a result of the accumulation of unrepaired cellular and molecular damage. This fact is well accepted; for example, Kirkwood[1] reviewed several maintenance and repair mechanisms involved in this process of accumulation (eg, somatic mutation theory, mitochondrial theory, altered proteins theory, network theories of aging). These theories point to the complexity of the networks and the stochastic nature of the many pathways that lead to damage. The theories also make clear that various repair mechanisms exist, which means that change with aging is not always deteriorative; improvement is also possible. This multidimensionality of change also contributes to the complexity of the aging process.

As people age, they accumulate deficits that are eventually manifested as frailty, disease, or disability. An important area of inquiry involves the extent to which subcellular deficit accumulation gives rise to the deficits that are visible clinically or by test procedures. In the progression from molecular damage to cellular damage and from cellular damage to tissues and then to organs, almost all adult-onset illnesses become more common with age, even if the role of age alone causing illness remains disputed.[1] Even though all illnesses become more common as people age, most older adults are fit and do not need or receive the specialized care of geriatricians. However, those who are

The research on frailty has been supported by the Canadian Institutes of Health Research and by the Fountain Innovation Fund of the Queen Elizabeth II Health Sciences Foundation. Professor Kenneth Rockwood receives career support through the Dalhousie Medical Research Foundation as the Kathryn Allen Weldon Professor of Alzheimer Research. The Canada-China Collaboration is funded jointly by the Canadian Institutes for Health Research and the National Natural Science Foundation of China. This article is written as part of that collaboration.
Division of Geriatric Medicine, Dalhousie University, Halifax, Room 1421, 5955 Veterans' Memorial Lane, Nova Scotia B3H 2E1, Canada
* Corresponding author.
E-mail address: Kenneth.Rockwood@Dal.Ca

frail would benefit from such care. This article considers the nature and operationalization of frailty and the role of complexity of frailty in the practice of geriatric medicine.

DEFINING FRAILTY CONCEPTUALLY AND OPERATIONALLY

There is a fair degree of consensus that frailty is an attribute of aged people who are at an increased risk of adverse health outcomes (including death) as a consequence of a diminished ability to respond to stress.[2] The authors would add that this diminished ability to respond to stress can be conceived of as a loss of redundancy, which arises as a consequence of the accumulation of multiple deficits.[3]

Many other contributions in this issue focus on the popular definition proposed and tested in the Cardiovascular Health Study in the United States and known as the phenotypic definition of frailty.[4] That study defined frailty by the occurrence of at least 3 of the following 5 deficits in an individual: slow walking speed, impaired grip strength, a self-report of declining activity levels, unintended weight loss, or exhaustion. The approach thus classified people as frail (3 or more deficits), prefrail (1 or 2 deficits), or robust (none of the deficits present). Although items have been combined by some in an index (from 0–5), generally degrees of frailty are not graded by this approach, for which it has been criticized. The phenotypic definition, in aiming to define a clinically recognizable group of people, also defines a frailty essence and excludes characteristics (such as disability, or complex comorbidity) that can be addressed using those constructs. Although none of the individual deficits are weighted, it has been suggested that mobility slowing is the key.[5]

The phenotypic definition finds its theoretical rationale in a "cycle of frailty." By this account, frailty gives rise to the so-called loss of physiologic reserve. The loss of reserve is itself otherwise unmeasured, so that the frailty characteristics serve as surrogates for this diminution in adaptive capacity. The phenotypic approach to frailty is the most widely studied approach, and in a variety of settings, this approach has been shown to correlate both with the risk of adverse outcomes and with many important clinical parameters.[6,7]

In addition to the phenotypic and other approaches, frailty is considered as an at-risk state caused by the age-associated accumulation of deficits.[8] A method has been proposed for how a frailty index can be derived from existing health databases by proposing criteria for deficits and procedures for counting deficits.[9] We count deficits as a whole range of health problems, which come in many forms: symptoms, signs, laboratory abnormalities, diseases, and disabilities. These features are clinically recognizable, and each represents an insult that has been insufficiently repaired and is referred to as a deficit. On average, people accumulate deficits as they age, but a challenge to understanding an essential property such as frailty is that people accumulate neither the same deficits nor the deficits at the same rate. One approach to this heterogeneity is to search for a small number of essential features that people who are at risk have in common. We have taken the opposite approach, in that we count deficits with little regard to their nature and studied instead whether the number (more particularly, the proportion) of deficits that people have defines their risk state. Our findings to now are that the number of deficits is important: the more deficits individuals accumulate, the more they are at risk of an adverse health outcome, that is, with more deficits, they are at more risk and so are more frail. In this sense, deficit accumulation is indistinguishable from the loss of physiologic reserve because it is the basis for this loss, and in systems engineering terms this loss is referred to as loss of redundancy.

As a first step, counting what is wrong needs to be standardized in some way. To date, the best way to count and standardize accumulated deficits is to combine them in an index. A convenient way for geriatricians to record and count deficits is to use the information gathered as part of a routine comprehensive geriatric assessment (CGA). We refer to the frailty index so constructed[10,11] as the frailty index based on a comprehensive geriatric assessment (FI-CGA). The total number of items that can be used in a frailty index is considered to be 80, for example, assuming that the maximum number of diagnoses is 15 and the maximum number of medications is 20.

Clearly, sometimes more than these numbers can be found, but for the most part, this is a reasonable assumption. How to score the effect of medications remains under investigation. At present, the approach is to count medications as deficits: 0 to 5 medications, no deficit; 5 to 7, 1 deficit; and an additional deficit is added for every 3 medications added after 7 medications for a maximum medication deficit count of 5. The latest version of a standard 1-page form to make up the FI-CGA is presented in **Fig. 1.** This version of the CGA form also includes 10 items that can be used to make up a social vulnerability index.[12] Although the list might seem daunting to non-geriatricians, specialists can recognize elements that are key to gaining a full understanding of a patient's health.

For any individual, a frailty index score based on CGA is calculated as the number of deficits that they have, divided by the total number of deficits that were considered, for example, 80. For example, a woman with diabetes, peptic ulcer disease, osteoarthritis, hypothyroidism, osteoporosis, and obesity (5 deficits), who takes 7 medications (1 deficit); needs help with banking, shopping, and transportation (3 deficits); complains of anxiety; rates her health as only fair; and seems poorly motivated to change her health status (2 deficits) would have 11 deficits. Therefore, her frailty index score would be the 11 deficits she has, divided by the 80 deficits that were considered, that is, an FI-CGA score of $11/80 = 0.14$.

A frailty index can be generated from almost any set of health-related variables, as long as a few criteria are met.[9] The criteria for an item to be considered as a deficit are that the item needs to be acquired, age-associated, and associated with an adverse outcome and should not saturate too early. The last criterion means that the proportion of people who have the deficit should not be close to 100% because the deficit is uninformative at that point. An example would be nocturia in men. Although nocturia is age associated, interrupts sleep, and is a deficit, the problem is common, typically seen in more than 90% of men older than 75 years.

Just as the FI-CGA mixes patient self-report with physician assessment and laboratory and other measurement data, we have evaluated several samples, which have used only self-report, almost all objective data, or some combination. Strikingly, in studies with more than 33,000 people from Canada, Australia, the United States, and Sweden, deficits accumulated exponentially with age, with an average relative rate of approximately 3% per annum on a log scale (**Fig. 2**).[13] In these studies, different variables were used in different datasets and the different datasets typically used variables that were not always overlapping, that is, different variables (we did not always consider the same variables) or even the same number of variables (we constructed frailty indices using 20–130 variables) were considered in different datasets.[14–16] Across datasets, increasing values of the frailty index are highly associated with an increased risk of death (**Fig. 3**). When both frailty index and age are combined in a multivariable model, in each case, the former has better predicted mortality than the latter. This difference remained even though the items that were counted in the frailty index were not the same each time. We consider this fact to be the evidence that the idea of frailty in relation to deficit accumulation is robust. In contrast to the traditional emphasis on exact duplication of instruments from one sample to the next, it seems that at a group level if not at the individual level (for individuals it is

Comprehensive Geriatric Assessment
Division of Geriatric Medicine, Dalhousie University

○ **Cognitive Status** — □ WNL □ Dementia MMSE: _____ □ CIND/MCI □ Delirium FAST: _____ Chief lifelong occupation: _____ Education (years): _____

○ **Emotional** — □ WNL □ ↓Mood □ Depression □ Anxiety □ Fatigue □ Other

○ **Motivation** — □ High □ Usual □ Low **Health Attitude** □ Excellent □ Good □ Fair □ Poor □ Couldn't say

○ **Communication** — Speech □ WNL □ Impaired Hearing □ WNL □ Impaired Vision □ WNL □ Impaired

○ **Strength** — □ WNL □ Weak Upper: PROXIMAL DISTAL Lower: PROXIMAL DISTAL

○ **Mobility** — Transfer: IND ASST DEP / IND ASST DEP; Walking: IND ASST DEP / IND ASST DEP; AID

○ **Balance** — Balance: IND IMPAIRED / IND IMPAIRED; Falls: N Y Number___ / N Y Number___

○ **Elimination** — Bowel: CONT CONSTIP INCONT / CONT CONSTIP INCONT; Bladder: CONT CATHETER INCONT / CONT CATHETER INCONT

○ **Nutrition** — Weight: GOOD UNDER OVER OBESE / STABLE LOSS GAIN; Appetite: WNL FAIR POOR / WNL FAIR POOR

○ **ADLs** — Feeding I A D / I A D; Bathing I A D / I A D; Dressing I A D / I A D; Toileting I A D / I A D

○ **IADLs** — Cooking I A D; Cleaning I A D; Shopping I A D; Medications I A D; Driving I A D; Banking I A D (baseline / current)

BASELINE (two weeks ago) / CURRENT (today) / NOTES

○ **Sleep** — □ Normal □ Disrupted □ Daytime drowsiness **Socially Engaged** □ Freq. □ Occ. □ Not

○ **Social** — □ Married □ Divorced □ Widowed □ Single; Lives: □ Alone □ Spouse □ Other; Home: □ House (levels___) □ Steps (Number___) □ Apartment □ Assisted living □ Nursing home □ Other; Supports: □ Informal □ HCNS □ Other □ None ○ Req. more support; Caregiver Relationship: □ Spouse □ Sibling □ Offspring □ Other; Caregiver stress: □ None □ Low □ Moderate □ High □ Advance directive in place? Caregiver occupation: (CG)

ACTION REQUIRED (check appropriate circles)

Problems: Med adjust req. Associated Medications: (*mark meds started in hospital with an asterisk)
1 RFR ○
2 ○
3 ○
4 ○
5 ○
6 ○
7 ○
8 ○
9 ○
10 ○

Patient contact: (Pt.) □ Inpatient □ Clinic □ GDH □ NH □ Outreach □ Home □ Assisted living □ ER □ Other
How many months since last well?
Current Frailty Score:
Scale	Pt.	CG
1. Very fit		
2. Well		
3. Well? Rx'd co-morbid disease		
4. Apparently vulnerable		
5. Mildly frail		
6. Moderately frail		
7. Severely frail		
8. Very severly frail		
9. Terminally ill		

Assessor/Physician: _____ Date: _____ YYYY/MM/DD

Fig. 1. FI-CGA form. (*Courtesy of* Geriatric Medicine Research Unit, Dalhousie University, Halifax, Nova Scotia.)

always important to know exactly what is wrong), the exact nature of a given deficit in relation to a person's state of health is less important than the deficit count. This approach has been confirmed by several independent studies.[17–21]

One intriguing but generally consistent finding from these analyses is that, at any given age, on average, women have more deficits than men. But if frailty is related to vulnerability risk, women are not frailer than men because for any given level of deficit accumulation, the mortality rate is higher in men than women. In other words, although women have more deficits than men, on average, they tolerate the deficits better. The biologic basis for this better toleration by women has yet to be established, but the finding is robust and implies a system effect.

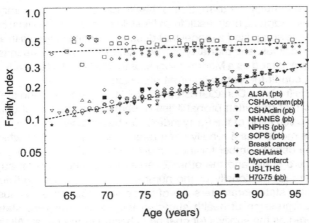

Fig. 2. The relationship between deficit accumulation and age. The lower line is the mean slope of deficit accumulation from surveys of community-dwelling people in 4 Western countries (Australia, Canada, the United States, and Sweden). The slope increases at about 0.03 per year. Note the log scale for the value of the frailty index. The upper line shows the relationship between the mean value of the frailty index and age for clinical and institutionalized samples. Note that the slope for those samples is close to 0, that is, these groups are, on average, so impaired that they cannot withstand another deficit, which is why no more deficits accumulate. (*From* Mitnitski A, Song X, Skoog I, et al. Relative fitness and frailty of elderly men and women in developed countries and their relationship with mortality. J Am Geriatr Soc 2005;53:2184–9; with permission.)

Change in the Frailty Index

It is well known that health generally does not improve with age. Deficits accumulate and this is reflected in the age-specific elevation of the trajectories of the frailty index. The trajectories can vary significantly within a group of individuals, reflecting the differences in each individual's aging rate. Individual trajectories can change in any

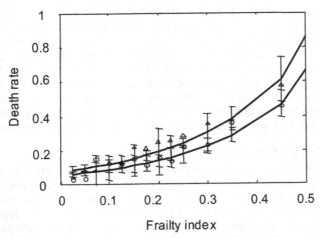

Fig. 3. The relationship between frailty index and mortality. Note that at all levels of the frailty index, deficit accumulation is more lethal for men than women. Triangles represent men and circles represent women.

direction, at least in the short term, that is, health can deteriorate or improve. Health improvement, for example, may result from lifestyle changes or medical interventions. Therefore, we have suggested a model that describes health changes in all directions: improvements, declines, and mortality.[22,23] We have developed a stochastic model of such changes considered as a Markov process and found that a relatively simple Poisson distribution can fit the data with great precision.

Our first results from the Canadian Study of Health and Aging, using the 5-year transitions, showed that transition probabilities of changes in the deficit count (which is fundamental to calculation of the frailty index) can be represented by a modified Poisson model. This model has 4 readily interpretable parameters, 2 of which represent transitions in the deficit number for those individuals who had no deficits at baseline (the so-called zero state) and the other 2 represent the incremental adjustment for these parameters proportionally to the number of deficits these individuals had at baseline. The zero state parameters are of particular importance because they indicate how the progression of health starts; in this sense, the zero state outcomes can be considered as the survival (or change in health) of the fittest. All these parameters can be easily adjusted for covariates. The model allows simultaneous estimation of the changes occurring as the individual improves, remains stable, declines, and eventually dies. Our preliminary results obtained in the Canadian Study of Health and Aging over 2 consecutive 5-year intervals were replicated in 2 different datasets: the National Population Health Survey (Canada) over 5 consecutive 2-year intervals[23] and Swedish birth cohort data (Gothenburg H-70 study).[24] In addition, this model of stochastic transitions was found to be equally applicable to cognitive changes[25,26] and was extended to address how exercise levels might affect such transitions. It was found that those who exercise regularly not only increase their survival chances but also improve or at least avoid deterioration of their cognitive functions. Finally, the same transition model was applied to social vulnerability, and the results were similar. This suggests that the model of health transitions has the power to not only predict the changes in health in any direction but also support analysis of the factors that might modify such changes.[27]

The high fit of the stochastic model of transitions supports the view that change generally happens gradually and depends on both the background and the individual state. Rapid change in the frailty index is often seen in people in the years before death. In fact, it seems that death of an individual can be better predicted based on the recent frailty index than on the review of past index values. Furthermore, review of the cumulative deficits over a long term may provide a better picture of the aging process and serve as a better predictor of death in the short term than does chronologic age. In other words, as people age, the accumulation of deficits accelerates, and this acceleration may be more useful in prediction than the individual's age. It is also clear that some people accumulate more deficits than others; for example, in the Canadian Study on Health and Aging, heavy smokers accumulated more deficits than nonsmokers.[28]

Frailty and "Biologic Age"

Given that deficit accumulation is so highly correlated with the risk of death, it is possible to view deficit accumulation as an estimate of biologic age. Consider 2 people, A and B, of the same chronologic age, for example, 78 years (**Fig. 4**). At 78 years, the mean value of the frailty index is 0.16. Person A has a frailty index value of 0.26 that is higher than the mean value by 0.1 corresponding to the mean value of the frailty index at age 93 years. In essence, person A has the life expectancy of a 93 years old; thus, although chronologically 78 years old, person A can be considered to be biologically 93 years old. By contrast, person B has a frailty index value of 0.1 that is lower than the mean value by

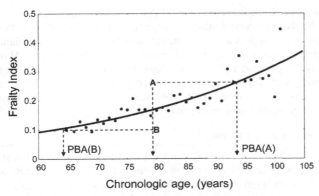

Fig. 4. Frailty and biologic age versus chronologic age.

0.06 corresponding to the mean value of the frailty index at age 63 years. In essence, person B has the life expectancy of a 63 years old; thus, although chronologically 78 years old, person B can be considered to be biologically 63 years old. Since we proposed this approach to the measurement of biologic age, 2 other groups have confirmed that the high correlation between mortality and deficit accumulation allows this approach to be considered further.[14,15,17]

Implications for Geriatric Medicine

We have proposed that frailty can be defined by deficit accumulation. One of the implications of this approach is that frailty can be considered as a complex phenomenon, and by acknowledging its complexity, we have shown that frailty has characteristic properties. Similarly, we propose that frailty can be embraced clinically, drawing on lessons from other undertakings in which complexity must be addressed. In the airline industry, for example, complexity is addressed through standard operating procedures and safety checks and identified through pattern recognition.[29] Each of these responses has so far been somewhat less formally developed in medicine. Although pattern recognition is crucial for clinical decision making, organization of information to facilitate pattern recognition is less well developed as a management strategy. As part of our strategic response to addressing the complexity of frailty, our group has focused on pattern recognition as a critical dimension of the definition and management of frailty.

Another common response to addressing the complexity of patients' needs and improving their care is the use of CGA.[30] Through assessment of general health (comorbidity), function, cognition, mood and motivation, the special senses, nutrition and medications, this tool facilitates identification of health issues and the appropriate intervention and follow-up for them. As part of a comprehensive management plan, CGA also supports continued independence and improved quality of life for an individual, in association with reduced medical costs.[31] Better patient care results from the acknowledgment of and focus on the complexity of frailty.

Other implications arise from considering the complexity of frailty. Frail elderly people can be viewed as complex systems on the brink of failure. As with other complex systems, failure generally begins with the highest-order functions. In the case of people, failure includes higher-order processing, walking upright, and planned social interaction. Failure of these high-level functions may result in delirium, falls, impaired function, and social withdrawal. These presentations have been described in the past as atypical but may in fact be typical of the frail elderly person.[32]

Although these presentations are typical in frail elderly people, there is variation in the grades of frailty and even limited changes in the number of deficits can lead to different prognoses. There is a strong correlation (0.8) between the clinical descriptions of the clinical frailty scale and the grades of the frailty index. Although some may question distinguishing between the "severe" and "very severe" frailty, there is a clear difference and those scoring at the very severe level have an accelerated risk of death. Individuals with a frailty index score greater than 0.55 have a median survival rate that is much lower than the median.

Frailty in Relation to Social Vulnerability

Social vulnerability, like frailty, has been easy to recognize clinically but has been the subject of debate over how it can best be operationalized. For example, social determinants of frailty have been discussed, and akin to the frailty index, a social vulnerability index has been proposed.[12] This index is based on social deficits drawn from a variety of indicators taken from theories such as social capital, social networks, social engagement, and social cohesion. Social vulnerability and frailty are related; greater social vulnerability is related to mortality in the elderly.

SUMMARY

Many older people are frail and have multiple diseases, disabilities, and other deficits that increase the likelihood of adverse outcomes. The complexity of their situations and variations in their deficit accumulation result in significant challenges for clinicians. The tendency is to attempt to precisely assess and provide individuals with detailed information on each deficit. In the past, providing such information has been perceived as more important than simply knowing how many deficits a person may have. However, the frailty index suggests that when deficits accumulate, it is the quantity of deficits that may be most significant in providing appropriate care. The specific details around existing deficits, or any new deficit that is identified, should not be foremost in the clinician's mind. Rather, each new deficit should be considered as part of the complex total picture.

Geriatricians have the opportunity to continuously improve the care of the elderly as more light is shed on the complexity of frailty. Acknowledging and accepting each person's "big picture" that includes a multitude of social and medical needs allow clinicians to provide more comprehensive treatment that prevents inappropriate efforts to dissect each issue and deal with it separately.

REFERENCES

1. Kirkwood TB. Understanding the odd science of aging. Cell 2006;120:437–47.
2. Abellan van Kan G, Rolland Y, Bergman H, et al. The I.A.N.A Task Force on frailty assessment of older people in clinical practice. J Nutr Health Aging 2008;12:29–37.
3. Lally F, Crome P. Understanding frailty. Postgrad Med J 2007;83:16–20.
4. Fried LP, Tangen CM, Walston J, et al. Frailty in older adults: evidence for a phenotype. J Gerontol A Biol Sci Med Sci 2001;56:M146–56.
5. Rothman MD, Leo-Summers L, Gill TM. Prognostic significance of potential frailty criteria. J Am Geriatr Soc 2008;56:2211–6.
6. Leng SX, Xue QL, Tian J, et al. Inflammation and frailty in older women. J Am Geriatr Soc 2007;55:864–71.
7. Hubbard RE, O'Mahony MS, Calver BL, et al. Nutrition, inflammation, and leptin levels in aging and frailty. J Am Geriatr Soc 2008;56:279–84.

8. Mitnitski AB, Mogilner AJ, Rockwood K. Accumulation of deficits as a proxy measure of aging. ScientificWorldJournal 2001;1:323–36.
9. Searle SD, Mitnitski A, Gahbauer EA, et al. A standard procedure for creating a frailty index. BMC Geriatr 2008;8:24.
10. Jones DM, Song X, Rockwood K. Operationalizing a frailty index from a standardized comprehensive geriatric assessment. J Am Geriatr Soc 2004;52:1929–33.
11. Jones D, Song X, Mitnitski A, et al. Evaluation of a frailty index based on a comprehensive geriatric assessment in a population based study of elderly Canadians. Aging Clin Exp Res 2005;17:465–71.
12. Andrew MK, Mitnitski AB, Rockwood K. Social vulnerability, frailty and mortality in elderly people. PLoS ONE 2008;3:e2232.
13. Mitnitski A, Song X, Skoog I, et al. Relative fitness and frailty of elderly men and women in developed countries and their relationship with mortality. J Am Geriatr Soc 2005;53:2184–9.
14. Kulminski AM, Ukraintseva SV, Kulminskaya IV, et al. Cumulative deficits better characterize susceptibility to death in elderly people than phenotypic frailty: lessons from the Cardiovascular Health Study. J Am Geriatr Soc 2008;56:898–903.
15. Woo J, Tang NL, Suen E, et al. Telomeres and frailty. Mech Ageing Dev 2008;129:642–8.
16. Rockwood K, Mitnitski A. Frailty in relation to the accumulation of deficits. J Gerontol A Biol Sci Med Sci 2007;62:722–7.
17. Goggins WB, Woo J, Sham A, et al. Frailty index as a measure of biological age in a Chinese population. J Gerontol A Biol Sci Med Sci 2005;60:1046–51.
18. Kulminski AM, Ukraintseva SV, Culminskaya IV, et al. Cumulative deficits and physiological indices as predictors of mortality and long life. J Gerontol A Biol Sci Med Sci 2008;63:1053–9.
19. Kulminski AM, Arbeev KG, Ukraintseva SV, et al. Changes in health status among participants of the Framingham Heart Study from the 1960s to the 1990s: application of an index of cumulative deficits. Ann Epidemiol 2008;18:696–701.
20. Kulminski A, Ukraintseva SV, Akushevich I, et al. Accelerated accumulation of health deficits as a characteristic of aging. Exp Gerontol 2007;42:963–70.
21. Gu D, Dupre ME, Sautter J, et al. Frailty and mortality among Chinese at advanced ages. J Gerontol B Psychol Sci Soc Sci 2009;64:279–89.
22. Mitnitski A, Bao L, Rockwood K. Going from bad to worse: a stochastic model of transitions in deficit accumulation, in relation to mortality. Mech Ageing Dev 2006;127:490–3.
23. Mitnitski A, Song X, Rockwood K. Improvement and decline in health status from late middle age: modeling age-related changes in deficit accumulation. Exp Gerontol 2007;42:1109–15.
24. Mitnitski A, Bao L, Skoog I, et al. A cross-national study of transitions in deficit counts in two birth cohorts: implications for modeling ageing. Exp Gerontol 2007;42(3):241–6.
25. Mitnitski A, Rockwood K. Transitions in cognitive test scores over 5 and 10 years in elderly people: evidence for a model of age-related deficit accumulation. BMC Geriatr 2008;8:3.
26. Middleton LE, Mitnitski A, Fallah N, et al. Changes in cognition and mortality in relation to exercise in late life: a population based study. PLoS One 2008;3(9):e3124.

27. Fallah N, Mitnitski A, Middleton L, et al. Modeling the impact of sex on how exercise is associated with cognitive changes and death in older Canadians. Neuroepidemiology 2009;33(1):47–54.
28. Hubbard RE, Searle SD, Mitnitski A, et al. Effect of smoking on the accumulation of deficits, frailty and survival in older adults: a secondary analysis from the Canadian Study of Health and Aging. J Nutr Health Aging 2009;13(5): 468–72.
29. Hales B, Terblanche M, Fowler R, et al. Improving patient care: the benefits of medical checklists. Int J Qual Health Care 2008;20:22–30.
30. Rockwood K, Silvius J, Fox RA. Comprehensive geriatric assessment. Helping your elderly patients maintain functional well-being. Postgrad Med 1998;103: 247–64.
31. Stuck AE, Siu AL, Wieland GD, et al. Comprehensive geriatric assessment: a meta-analysis of controlled trials. Lancet 1993;342(8878):1032–6.
32. Jarrett PG, Rockwood K, Carver D, et al. Illness presentations in elderly patients. Arch Intern Med 1995;155:1060–4.

The Biology of Aging and Frailty

Neal S. Fedarko, PhD

KEYWORDS

• Frailty • Aging • Apoptosis • Senescence • Inflammation

In developing and validating the concept of frailty as a geriatric syndrome, it has been necessary to distinguish the clinical expression of frailty from normal age-related changes and other age-related disease pathologies. Fried and colleagues[1–5] have provided a framework for excluding potentially confounding disease and a working clinical tool to diagnose frailty, and they have shown associations between frailty and other pathophysiologies. However, investigating the underlying biologic basis for the geriatric syndrome of frailty by studying basic homeostatic pathways and mechanisms has not proceeded at the same rate. The following article provides an overview of the homeostatic pathways emphasized in research on aging and explains how this science may help to stimulate frailty research.

NORMAL AGING

Aging can be defined as the decline and deterioration of functional properties at the cellular, tissue, and organ level. This loss of functional properties yields a loss of homeostasis and a decreased adaptability to internal and external stress, increasing vulnerability to disease and mortality.[6] Aging is a breakdown in maintenance of specific molecular structures and pathways, a loss of homeostasis, and a failure in homeodynamics.[7] Homeodynamics refers to biologic systems that do not actively mandate stasis; instead, they dynamically reorganize and reset points of balance in response to internal and external change to maintain their functional capacity over time.

Individuals vary a great deal in the onset of the aging process and the rate and extent of its progression. Differences in the manifestations of aging reflect differences in functional capacity. Functional capacity is a direct measure of the ability of cells, tissues, and organ systems to operate properly/optimally and is influenced by genes and environment. Optimal cellular, organ, and organism operation reflects homeodynamic mechanisms and maintenance pathways. Mechanisms of maintenance include DNA repair, synthesis, and fidelity surveillance; detection and clearance of defective proteins

This work was supported in part by Grant No. AG000120 from the National Institutes of Health.
Division of Geriatric Medicine and Gerontology, Department of Medicine, Johns Hopkins University School of Medicine, Johns Hopkins University, 5501 Hopkins Bayview Circle, Baltimore, MD 21224, USA
E-mail address: ndarko@jhmi.edu

and lipids; clearance of defective organelles and cells; and defense against pathogens and injury. Many of the physiologic theories of aging are direct counterparts of these maintenance mechanisms (eg, DNA damage, error catastrophe, free-radical, mito-chondrial damage, and immunosenescence theories). These maintenance mecha-nisms, in turn, affect homeodynamics through the cellular responses of apoptosis, senescence, and repair and the systemic response of immune activation/inflammation. For example, when DNA damage is too great to be repaired, cells undergo apoptosis.[8] Cells can respond to free-radical damage to DNA by inducing senescence[9] or initiating apoptosis.[10] Oxidative damage and apoptosis are correlated negatively with the repair mechanism autophagy.[11] Proteins aberrantly modified with nonenzymatic glycation[12] or free radicals[13] can induce inflammation. Inflammation and immune responses resolve, in part, through targeted immune cell apoptosis.[14] In addition to critical telo-mere length, senescence can be triggered by oxidative stress[9,15] and protein glyca-tion/cross-links.[16,17] Hormones contribute to homeodynamics, in part, through modulation of apoptosis, senescence, and inflammation.[18–20]

FRAILTY

Frailty is a geriatric syndrome characterized by weakness, weight loss, and low activity and is associated with adverse health outcomes. Frailty manifests as age-related, bio-logic vulnerability to stressors and decreased physiologic reserves yielding a limited capacity to maintain homeostasis.[3] The validated and widely used 5-item frailty criteria for screening—self-reported exhaustion, slowed performance (by walking speed), weakness (by grip strength), unintentional weight loss (4.5 kg in the past year), and low physical activity[1]—are composite outcomes of multiple organ systems. The surrogate endpoint markers—elevated cytokines and chemokines[21–23]; reduced insulinlike growth factor 1(IGF-I), dehydroepiandrosterone sulfate, and leptin[24]; perturbed neutrophil, monocyte, and white blood cell distribution[25,26]—indicate multiple systems are dysregulated in frailty.

This definition of frailty (multisystem dysregulation yielding decreased physiologic reserves and increased vulnerability to stressors) has commonality to that of aging (loss of molecular/cellular functional properties yielding decreased adaptability to internal/external stress and increased vulnerability to disease and mortality). Both have a basis in loss of homeostasis, although with aging, the failure in homeodynamics is global, whereas with frailty, the failure in homeodynamics cycle around energy metabolism and neuromuscular changes. Because researchers have characterized frail elderly populations, the observed changes in functional performance and biomarker distribution are distinct from the corresponding age-related changes observed in nonfrail (normal) individuals.[1–4]

CELLULAR RESPONSES TO STRESSORS

For aging and frailty, loss of homeostasis results in an increased vulnerability to stressors. An organism's reaction to stressors involves the cellular responses of apoptosis, senescence, and repair. At the cellular level, stressors (eg, free radicals, DNA damage, cell injury/insult) challenge maintenance mechanisms (**Fig. 1**). The evolved cellular response, apoptosis, removes damaged/aberrant cells through controlled cell death; senescence alters their phenotype and blocks further prolifera-tion; and repair removes damaged proteins, lipids, and organelles and recycles constituent parts. Failure in these responses leads to transformed cells/neoplasms that can radically compromise organ function and survival. Dysregulation of these cellular responses can contribute to tissue pathology when, for example, increased

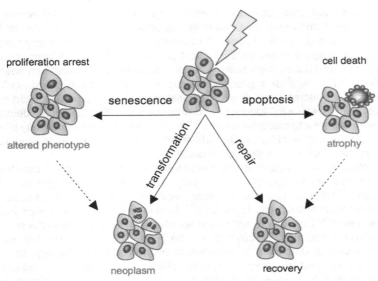

proliferation arrest

senescence

apoptosis

cell death

altered phenotype

transformation

repair

atrophy

neoplasm

recovery

Fig. 1. Cellular responses to stressors. Stressors (free radicals, DNA damage, nutrient or oxygen constriction, cell injury [represented by the *lightening bolt*]) challenge cellular homeostasis. The cellular response can be senescence, apoptosis, repair, or neoplastic transformation of the cell. Senescence, a tumor-suppressive response is associated with an altered secretory phenotype. The controlled cell death of apoptosis can also be tumor-suppressive, although many cells, especially immune cells, normally exit through apoptosis. Apoptosis can, however, yield tissue/organ atrophy. Repair enables recovery of homeostasis. In some cases, apoptosis is a precursor of repair and recovery (*dotted line* with *arrow*). Also, the senescent cell phenotype is sometimes a precursor/contributor to neoplasm formation and cancer progression.

apoptosis leads to tissue/organ atrophy or when expression of the senescent cell phenotype increases proinflammatory cytokine release. All these cellular responses have been implicated in normal aging and are discussed in greater detail in the following sections. The balance between apoptosis and senescence or the acceleration of either may well precipitate changes in multiple systems and, ultimately, in frailty and related late-life vulnerability.

Apoptosis

Apoptosis is an orderly process of cellular self-destruction, a process as crucial for survival of multicellular organisms as cell division. Apoptosis is important in embryogenesis: morphogenesis (eliminating excess cells, such as webbing between digits in embryos), selection (eliminating nonfunctional cells, as in neuronal pruning), immunity (eliminating dangerous cells, such as self-antigen recognizing cells), and organ size (eliminating excess cells).[27] Apoptosis is also important in adults in tissue remodeling (eliminating cells no longer needed, as in mammary gland involution after lactation), maintains organ size and function,[28] and eliminates damaged/dysfunctional cells.[29,30]

Apoptosis can be initiated by external signals that bind to physiologic receptors on cell surfaces or by intrinsic damage that propagates cytosolic signals. Both pathways converge with mitochondrial signals, which lead to a caspase cleavage cascade, which, in turn, results in the orderly proteolysis of proteins and DNA, the cross-linking of cell corpses, and their subsequent engulfment. Although death by necrosis and oncosis (ischemic cell death) invokes major inflammatory responses and collateral damage, apoptosis is a controlled cellular demolition with no inflammatory response. Key apoptosis steps (chromatin condensation, vesicle formation, and activity of hydrolytic enzymes) have a high energy demand and thus, apoptosis is an adenosine triphosphate (ATP)-dependent process.[31] Thus, at insufficient ATP levels, cells shift from apoptotic to necrotic cell death.[32] Consistent with this, an age-related decline in cellular ATP levels was found to promote necrotic fibroblast cell death over apoptosis in response to oxidative stress.[33] These molecular processes may stimulate chronic inflammation in older adults, which probably facilitates frailty and late-life decline through mechanisms discussed below.

As a sentinel homeodynamic cellular response, apoptosis can have pathophysiologic consequences for aging. For example, too much apoptosis can yield tissue degeneration,[34] whereas too little apoptosis allows dysfunctional cells to accumulate or differentiated immune cells to persist.[35] Evidence suggests that sarcopenia is apoptosis-driven.[36] Conversely, failures in apoptosis can contribute to the senescent cell phenotype as well as rogue cell proliferation.[37] It has been shown that apoptosis is an important cellular defense mechanism in maintaining genetic stability, and centenarians who have aged successfully possess cells that are more prone to apoptosis.[38] The proinflammatory marker interleukin 6 (IL-6) seems to be protective against apoptosis[39] and its serum levels are known to increase with increasing age[40] and have an inverse correlation with apoptosis.[41]

Senescence

Cellular senescence is a response of normal cells to potentially cancer-causing events. The term replicative senescence identifies the subset of senescent cells in which the arrest in proliferation is associated with the high number of cell divisions (the Hayflick and Moorhead[42] limit—typically between 40 and 60 cell divisions). The mechanism for replicative senescence involves each division resulting in a shortening of the telomere region of chromosomes, such that a cumulative critical length is reached that does not support the DNA replication machinery. Senescent cells exhibit an irreversible arrest of cell proliferation, an altered function, and in some cases, a resistance to apoptosis. Besides telomere shortening, inducers of senescence include DNA damage, oncogene expression, supermitogenic signals,[43] and telomere-independent pathways, which include cytoskeletal, interferon-related, IGF-related, mitogen-activated protein kinase, and oxidative stress pathways.[44] The arrest in proliferation is imposed and maintained on cells by the induction of cyclin-dependent kinase inhibitors p16 and p21 that implement cell-cycle arrest.[45] Cellular senescence is associated with typical phenotypic changes, such as enlarged morphology, activation of senescence-associated β-galactosidase, elevated expression of proteases, cell-cycle inhibitors, and proinflammatory cytokines.[43]

The contribution of cellular (replicative) senescence to organismal aging has been controversial, although increasingly; evidence seems to link cellular senescence to aging.[46,47] Senescent cells accumulate with age and at sites of age-related pathology.[47] The senescent phenotype (eg, secretion of IL-6) may contribute to the proinflammatory state observed in normal aging that is exacerbated in frailty.

Repair

The repair cellular response involves removal of damaged proteins/lipids and organelles and recycling of constituent components via the catabolic/degradative machinery of cells—proteasomes, lysosomes, and autophagosomes.[48] Proteasomes are large cellular protein complexes that degrade unnecessary or damaged proteins tagged with ubiquitin. Lysosomes are cellular organelles that fuse with vacuoles and dispense enzymes that degrade proteins, polysaccharides, nucleic acids, and lipids present in the vacuoles. Autophagosomes are involved in sequestering cytosolic components/organelles through phagophore formation, fusing the formed autophagosome with lysosomes, and degrading material by the lysosomal machinery (ie, autophagy). Normal cycling (flux) of these cellular catabolic vacuoles prevents the accumulation of damaged/aberrant molecular and cellular components.[49]

The removal and recycling phases of repair have gained considerable interest in research on aging. Conditions that modulate lifespan—mutations in the insulin/IGF-I signaling system, treatments that reduce the expression/activity of the transcription factor mammalian target of rapamycin (mTOR), and caloric restriction all increase autophagy.[49] Aging cells exhibit an increase in mitochondrial DNA mutations and a decline in mitochondrial function.[50] Also, free radical generation by damaged mitochondria increases. Autophagy normally maintains homeostasis through mitochondrial turnover. Dysregulation of autophagy,[51] proteasomes,[52] and lysosomes[53] have all been observed with increasing age. Thus, functional capacity to remove oxidized, cross-linked, and/or unfolded proteins, nucleic acids, lipids, and polysaccharides is impaired, and these products increase with age. Lipofuscin ("aging pigment") arises in lysosomes through the oxidation of unsaturated fatty acids through iron-generated free radicals. Lipofuscin is insoluble and refractile to cellular removal and recycling, accumulates with age, and may compromise organelle functional capacity by "overstuffing" organelles or diverting hydrolases and lipases away from their normal substrates.

SYSTEMIC RESPONSES TO STRESSORS: INFLAMMATION

Inflammation is a sentinel systemic response to stressors that plays a central role in the aging process in normal, healthy individuals.[54] The classic definition of inflammation refers to 5 cardinal signs: *calor* (heat), *dolor* (pain), *rubor* (redness), *tumor* (swelling), and *functio laesa* (loss of function). Inflammation modulates the cellular responses to stressors, and cellular responses can regulate components of the inflammatory response. Immunosenescence is the decline in the function of the adaptive immune system that occurs during aging that is associated with thymic involution, alterations in T-cell subsets, and reduction in antibody production. As adaptive immunity declines, innate immunity systems exhibit low-level but chronic activation that, with oxidative stress, leads to a low-level but chronic proinflammatory phenotype. A proinflammatory state may underlie several pathologies, including cancer,[55] cardiovascular disease,[56,57] diabetes mellitus,[58] osteoporosis,[59] rheumatoid arthritis,[60] and cognitive disorders, such as Alzheimer and Parkinson disease.[61] It is thought that these altered cytokines, in the local tissue microenvironment, perturb cellular functional capacity facilitating disease progression. "Inflammaging" is the term used to describe this proinflammatory state associated with aging,[62] which has also been termed molecular inflammation.[63,64]

Several studies have shown significant association of elevated IL-6 levels with frailty in older adults.[21,22,25,65,66] The altered inflammatory state observed in frailty may contribute to several frailty-associated pathologies. For example, proinflammatory cytokines affect the growth hormone/IGF-I axis.[67] "Sickness behavior" (fatigue, malaise, loss of interest in social activities, difficulty concentrating, and changes in sleep patterns) is triggered by the production of proinflammatory cytokines by macrophages and other cells of the innate immune system in response to immune

Table 1
Cellular and systemic response regulation by key transcription factors

	Transcription Factor			
Response	p53	Rb	NF-κB	FOXO
Apoptosis	↑[72]	↓[73]	↓[74]	↑[75]
Senescence	↑[76]	↑[45]	↑[77]	↑[78]
Repair/autophagy	↓[79]	↓[80]	↓[81]	↑[82]
Inflammation	↓[83]	↓[84]	↑[85]	↓[86]

The induction (↑) or repression (↓) of cellular and systemic responses by key transcription factors and the references supporting that assessment are given in parenthesis.

challenge.[68] The *cytokine hypothesis of depression* suggests that proinflammatory cytokines can act as neuromodulators—key factors in the (central) mediation of the behavioral, neuroendocrine, and neurochemical features of depressive disorders.[69,70] The central action of cytokines may also account for the hypothalamic-pituitary-adrenal (HPA) axial hyperactivity that is frequently observed in several age-related disorders, because proinflammatory cytokines disturb the negative feedback inhibition of circulating corticosteroids on the HPA axis.[71–86]

CROSS TALK BETWEEN CELLULAR RESPONSES AND INFLAMMATION

The tumor suppressors retinoblastoma protein (pRb), p53, and forkhead transcription factor (FOXO) are key modulators of apoptosis, senescence, and repair responses. The central transcription factor in inflammatory responses is nuclear factor kappaB (NF-κB). NF-κB also modulates apoptosis, senescence, and repair responses. The proteins p53, pRb, FOXO, and NF-κB are controlled by complex pathways involving upstream regulators, downstream effectors, and cytosolic inhibitors (for NF-κB) that regulate expression of other genes, modulate cell-cycle progression, and are crucial for allowing normal cells to sense and respond to apoptosis and senescence signals. These transcription factors have direct effects on increasing or decreasing cellular responses (**Table 1**).

Interaction between p53 and pRb is well known in their role in determining whether DNA damage can be repaired or whether apoptosis should occur.[87] Cross talk also occurs between p53 and FOXO[88] and pRb and NF-κB.[89] The communication between response regulators can be multileveled. For example, p53 acts in at least 2 stages of inflammation—as a general inhibitor of NF-κB-dependent transcription and, through an unknown mechanism, as a positive regulator of neutrophil clearance by macrophages.[90]

SUMMARY

The cellular responses of apoptosis, senescence, and repair and the systemic response of immune activation/inflammation have evolving roles in contributing to the aging phenotype. Homeostatic mechanisms effect change through these responses; thus, they are likely candidates for pathways that may contribute to the failure in homeodynamics seen in frailty. Dysregulation of apoptosis may contribute to the frailty traits of sarcopenia and weakness. Similarly, the cellular senescent phenotype, secreting proinflammatory cytokines, may contribute to the dysregulated inflammatory state seen in frailty. One can further speculate that deficits in repair in specific tissues (eg, muscle, nerves, bone) contribute to frailty. Facets of senescence, apoptosis, and repair response have yet to be carefully studied in the setting of frailty. It may be expected that the patterns observed in normal aging between these different cellular and systemic responses would be further perturbed or accelerated in the syndrome of frailty. Future investigations targeting these areas will provide the data necessary to test these hypotheses related to the biology of aging.

REFERENCES

1. Fried LP, Tangen CM, Walston J, et al. Frailty in older adults: evidence for a phenotype. J Gerontol A Biol Sci Med Sci 2001;56(3):M146–56.
2. Walston J, McBurnie MA, Newman A, et al. Frailty and activation of the inflammation and coagulation systems with and without clinical comorbidities: results from the Cardiovascular Health Study. Arch Intern Med 2002;162(20):2333–41.
3. Fried LP, Ferrucci L, Darer J, et al. Untangling the concepts of disability, frailty, and comorbidity: implications for improved targeting and care. J Gerontol A Biol Sci Med Sci 2004;59(3):255–63.
4. Bandeen-Roche K, Xue QL, Ferrucci L, et al. Phenotype of frailty: characterization in the women's health and aging studies. J Gerontol A Biol Sci Med Sci 2006; 61(3):262–6.
5. Chang SS, Weiss CO, Xue QL, et al. Patterns of comorbid inflammatory diseases in frail older women: the Women's Health and Aging Studies I and II. J Gerontol A Biol Sci Med Sci 2010;65(4):407–13.
6. Holliday R, Understanding ageing. Developmental and cell biology series; 30. Cambridge (UK); New York: Cambridge University Press; 1995. p. xiv, 207.
7. Lloyd D, Aon MA, Cortassa S. Why homeodynamics, not homeostasis? Scientific-WorldJournal 2001;1:133–45.
8. Roos WP, Kaina B. DNA damage-induced cell death by apoptosis. Trends Mol Med 2006;12(9):440–50.
9. Chen Q, Fischer A, Reagan JD, et al. Oxidative DNA damage and senescence of human diploid fibroblast cells. Proc Natl Acad Sci U S A 1995;92(10):4337–41.
10. Ozawa T. Oxidative damage and fragmentation of mitochondrial DNA in cellular apoptosis. Biosci Rep 1997;17(3):237–50.
11. Wohlgemuth SE, Seo AY, Marzetti E, et al. Skeletal muscle autophagy and apoptosis during aging: effects of calorie restriction and life-long exercise. Exp Gerontol 2010;45(2):138–48.
12. Ramasamy R, Vannucci SJ, Yan SS, et al. Advanced glycation end products and RAGE: a common thread in aging, diabetes, neurodegeneration, and inflammation. Glycobiology 2005;15(7):16R–28R.
13. Nabeshi H, Oikawa S, Inoue S, et al. Proteomic analysis for protein carbonyl as an indicator of oxidative damage in senescence-accelerated mice. Free Radic Res 2006;40(11):1173–81.
14. Marshall JC, Watson RW. Programmed cell death (apoptosis) and the resolution of systemic inflammation. Can J Surg 1997;40(3):169–74.
15. von Zglinicki T. Role of oxidative stress in telomere length regulation and replicative senescence. Ann N Y Acad Sci 2000;908:99–110.
16. Nagaraj RH, Sell DR, Prabhakaram M, et al. High correlation between pentosidine protein crosslinks and pigmentation implicates ascorbate oxidation in human lens senescence and cataractogenesis. Proc Natl Acad Sci U S A 1991;88(22):10257–61.
17. Ravelojaona V, Robert AM, Robert L. Expression of senescence-associated beta-galactosidase (SA-beta-Gal) by human skin fibroblasts, effect of advanced

glycation end-products and fucose or rhamnose-rich polysaccharides. Arch Gerontol Geriatr 2008;48(2):151–4.

18. Evans-Storms RB, Cidlowski JA. Regulation of apoptosis by steroid hormones. J Steroid Biochem Mol Biol 1995;53(1–6):1–8.

19. Hertoghe T. The "multiple hormone deficiency" theory of aging: is human senescence caused mainly by multiple hormone deficiencies? Ann N Y Acad Sci 2005; 1057:448–65.

20. Roubenoff R. Molecular basis of inflammation: relationships between catabolic cytokines, hormones, energy balance, and muscle. JPEN J Parenter Enteral Nutr 2008;32(6):630–2.

21. Leng S, Chaves P, Koenig K, et al. Serum interleukin-6 and hemoglobin as physiological correlates in the geriatric syndrome of frailty: a pilot study. J Am Geriatr Soc 2002;50(7):1268–71.

22. De Martinis M, Franceschi C, Monti D, et al. Inflammation markers predicting frailty and mortality in the elderly. Exp Mol Pathol 2006;80(3):219–27.

23. Qu T, Yang H, Walston JD, et al. Upregulated monocytic expression of CXC chemokine ligand 10 (CXCL-10) and its relationship with serum interleukin-6 levels in the syndrome of frailty. Cytokine 2009;46(3):319–24.

24. Hubbard RE, O'Mahony MS, Calver BL, et al. Plasma esterases and inflammation in ageing and frailty. Eur J Clin Pharmacol 2008;64(9):895–900.

25. Leng SX, Xue QL, Tian J, et al. Inflammation and frailty in older women. J Am Geriatr Soc 2007;55(6):864–71.

26. Leng SX, Xue QL, Tian J, et al. Associations of neutrophil and monocyte counts with frailty in community-dwelling disabled older women: results from the Women's Health and Aging Studies I. Exp Gerontol 2009;44(8):511–6.

27. Haanen C, Vermes I. Apoptosis: programmed cell death in fetal development. Eur J Obstet Gynecol Reprod Biol 1996;64(1):129–33.

28. Mondello C, Scovassi AI. Apoptosis: a way to maintain healthy individuals. Subcell Biochem 2010;50:307–23.

29. Muradian K, Schachtschabel DO. The role of apoptosis in aging and age-related disease: update. Z Gerontol Geriatr 2001;34(6):441–6.

30. Pollack M, Phaneuf S, Dirks A, et al. The role of apoptosis in the normal aging brain, skeletal muscle, and heart. Ann N Y Acad Sci 2002;959:93–107.

31. Kass GE, Eriksson JE, Weis M, et al. Chromatin condensation during apoptosis requires ATP. Biochem J 1996;318(Pt 3):749–52.

32. Richter C, Schweizer M, Cossarizza A, et al. Control of apoptosis by the cellular ATP level. FEBS Lett 1996;378(2):107–10.

33. Miyoshi N, Oubrahim H, Chock PB, et al. Age-dependent cell death and the role of ATP in hydrogen peroxide-induced apoptosis and necrosis. Proc Natl Acad Sci U S A 2006;103(6):1727–31.

34. Adams JD, Mukherjee SK, Klaidman LK, et al. Apoptosis and oxidative stress in the aging brain. Ann N Y Acad Sci 1996;786:135–51.

35. Gupta S. Molecular mechanisms of apoptosis in the cells of the immune system in human aging. Immunol Rev 2005;205:114–29.

36. Marzetti E, Leeuwenburgh C. Skeletal muscle apoptosis, sarcopenia and frailty at old age. Exp Gerontol 2006;41(12):1234–8.

37. Hsu HC, Scott DK, Mountz JD. Impaired apoptosis and immune senescence - cause or effect? Immunol Rev 2005;205:130–46.

38. Franceschi C, Monti D, Scarfi MR, et al. Genomic instability and aging. Studies in centenarians (successful aging) and in patients with Down's syndrome (accelerated aging). Ann N Y Acad Sci 1992;663:4–16.

39. Biffl WL, Moore EE, Moore FA, et al. Interleukin-6 delays neutrophil apoptosis. Arch Surg 1996;131(1):24–9 [discussion: 9–30].
40. Giuliani N, Sansoni P, Girasole G, et al. Serum interleukin-6, soluble interleukin-6 receptor and soluble gp130 exhibit different patterns of age- and menopause-related changes. Exp Gerontol 2001;36(3):547–57.
41. Kovalovich K, Li W, DeAngelis R, et al. Interleukin-6 protects against Fas-mediated death by establishing a critical level of anti-apoptotic hepatic proteins FLIP, Bcl-2, and Bcl-xL. J Biol Chem 2001;276(28):26605–13.
42. Hayflick L, Moorhead PS. The serial cultivation of human diploid cell strains. Exp Cell Res 1961;25:585–621.
43. Muller M. Cellular senescence: molecular mechanisms, in vivo significance, and redox considerations. Antioxid Redox Signal 2009;11(1):59–98.
44. Fridman AL, Tainsky MA. Critical pathways in cellular senescence and immortalization revealed by gene expression profiling. Oncogene 2008;27(46): 5975–87.
45. Ohtani N, Yamakoshi K, Takahashi A, et al. The p16INK4a-RB pathway: molecular link between cellular senescence and tumor suppression. J Med Invest 2004; 51(3–4):146–53.
46. Campisi J. Cellular senescence and apoptosis: how cellular responses might influence aging phenotypes. Exp Gerontol 2003;38(1–2):5–11.
47. Jeyapalan JC, Sedivy JM. Cellular senescence and organismal aging. Mech Ageing Dev 2008;129(7–8):467–74.
48. Korolchuk VI, Menzies FM, Rubinsztein DC. Mechanisms of cross-talk between the ubiquitin-proteasome and autophagy-lysosome systems. FEBS Lett 2010; 584(7):1393–8.
49. Vellai T, Takacs-Vellai K, Sass M, et al. The regulation of aging: does autophagy underlie longevity? Trends Cell Biol 2009;19(10):487–94.
50. Wallace DC. A mitochondrial paradigm of metabolic and degenerative diseases, aging, and cancer: a dawn for evolutionary medicine. Annu Rev Genet 2005;39: 359–407.
51. Cuervo AM, Bergamini E, Brunk UT, et al. Autophagy and aging: the importance of maintaining "clean" cells. Autophagy 2005;1(3):131–40.
52. Chondrogianni N, Gonos ES. Proteasome dysfunction in mammalian aging: steps and factors involved. Exp Gerontol 2005;40(12):931–8.
53. Chondrogianni N, Fragoulis EG, Gonos ES. Protein degradation during aging: the lysosome-, the calpain- and the proteasome-dependent cellular proteolytic systems. Biogerontology 2002;3(1–2):121–3.
54. Stout RD, Suttles J. Immunosenescence and macrophage functional plasticity: dysregulation of macrophage function by age-associated microenvironmental changes. Immunol Rev 2005;205:60–71.
55. Aggarwal BB, Shishodia S, Sandur SK, et al. Inflammation and cancer: how hot is the link? Biochem Pharmacol 2006;72(11):1605–21.
56. Osiecki H. The role of chronic inflammation in cardiovascular disease and its regulation by nutrients. Altern Med Rev 2004;9(1):32–53.
57. Diomedi M, Leone G, Renna A. The role of chronic infection and inflammation in the pathogenesis of cardiovascular and cerebrovascular disease. Drugs Today (Barc) 2005;41(11):745–53.
58. Duncan BB, Schmidt MI. The epidemiology of low-grade chronic systemic inflammation and type 2 diabetes. Diabetes Technol Ther 2006;8(1):7–17.
59. Ginaldi L, Di Benedetto MC, De Martinis M. Osteoporosis, inflammation and ageing. Immun Ageing 2005;2:14.

60. Wong SH, Lord JM. Factors underlying chronic inflammation in rheumatoid arthritis. Arch Immunol Ther Exp (Warsz) 2004;52(6):379–88.
61. McGeer PL, McGeer EG. Inflammation and the degenerative diseases of aging. Ann N Y Acad Sci 2004;1035:104–16.
62. Giunta S. Is inflammaging an auto[innate]immunity subclinical syndrome? Immun Ageing 2006;3:12.
63. Chung HY, Kim HJ, Kim KW, et al. Molecular inflammation hypothesis of aging based on the anti-aging mechanism of calorie restriction. Microsc Res Tech 2002;59(4):264–72.
64. Chung HY, Cesari M, Anton S, et al. Molecular inflammation: underpinnings of aging and age-related diseases. Ageing Res Rev 2009;8(1):18–30.
65. Leng SX, Yang H, Walston JD. Decreased cell proliferation and altered cytokine production in frail older adults. Aging Clin Exp Res 2004;16(3):249–52.
66. Hubbard RE, O'Mahony MS, Calver BL, et al. Nutrition, inflammation, and leptin levels in aging and frailty. J Am Geriatr Soc 2008;56(2):279–84.
67. Johnson RW, Arkins S, Dantzer R, et al. Hormones, lymphohemopoietic cytokines and the neuroimmune axis. Comp Biochem Physiol A Physiol 1997;116(3): 183–201.
68. Dantzer R, Bluthe RM, Laye S, et al. Cytokines and sickness behavior. Ann N Y Acad Sci 1998;840:586–90.
69. Myint AM, Kim YK. Cytokine-serotonin interaction through IDO: a neurodegeneration hypothesis of depression. Med Hypotheses 2003;61(5–6):519–25.
70. Schiepers OJ, Wichers MC, Maes M. Cytokines and major depression. Prog Neuropsychopharmacol Biol Psychiatry 2005;29(2):201–17.
71. Porter RJ, Gallagher P, O'Brien JT. Effects of rapid tryptophan depletion on salivary cortisol in older people recovered from depression, and the healthy elderly. J Psychopharmacol 2007;21(1):71–5.
72. Harbour JW, Dean DC. Rb function in cell-cycle regulation and apoptosis. Nat Cell Biol 2000;2(4):E65–7.
73. Fridman JS, Lowe SW. Control of apoptosis by p53. Oncogene 2003;22(56): 9030–40.
74. Cardoso SM, Oliveira CR. Inhibition of NF-kB renders cells more vulnerable to apoptosis induced by amyloid beta peptides. Free Radic Res 2003;37(9): 967–73.
75. Jagani Z, Singh A, Khosravi-Far R. FoxO tumor suppressors and BCR-ABL-induced leukemia: a matter of evasion of apoptosis. Biochim Biophys Acta 2008;1785(1):63–84.
76. Wesierska-Gadek J, Ranftler C, Schmid G. Physiological ageing: role of p53 and PARP-1 tumor suppressors in the regulation of terminal senescence. J Physiol Pharmacol 2005;56(Suppl 2):77–88.
77. Bernard D, Gosselin K, Monte D, et al. Involvement of Rel/nuclear factor-kappaB transcription factors in keratinocyte senescence. Cancer Res 2004;64(2):472–81.
78. Kyoung Kim H, Kyoung Kim Y, Song IH, et al. Down-regulation of a forkhead transcription factor, FOXO3a, accelerates cellular senescence in human dermal fibroblasts. J Gerontol A Biol Sci Med Sci 2005;60(1):4–9.
79. Maiuri MC, Galluzzi L, Morselli E, et al. Autophagy regulation by p53. Curr Opin Cell Biol 2010;22(2):181–5.
80. Tracy K, Dibling BC, Spike BT, et al. BNIP3 is an RB/E2F target gene required for hypoxia-induced autophagy. Mol Cell Biol 2007;27(17):6229–42.
81. Copetti T, Bertoli C, Dalla E, et al. p65/RelA modulates BECN1 transcription and autophagy. Mol Cell Biol 2009;29(10):2594–608.

82. Zhao J, Brault JJ, Schild A, et al. Coordinate activation of autophagy and the pro-teasome pathway by FoxO transcription factor. Autophagy 2008;4(3):378–80.
83. Zheng SJ, Lamhamedi-Cherradi SE, Wang P, et al. Tumor suppressor p53 inhibits autoimmune inflammation and macrophage function. Diabetes 2005;54(5): 1423–8.
84. Ying L, Marino J, Hussain SP, et al. Chronic inflammation promotes retinoblastoma protein hyperphosphorylation and E2F1 activation. Cancer Res 2005;65(20): 9132–6.
85. Tak PP, Firestein GS. NF-kappaB: a key role in inflammatory diseases. J Clin Invest 2001;107(1):7–11.
86. Snoeks L, Weber CR, Wasland K, et al. Tumor suppressor FOXO3 participates in the regulation of intestinal inflammation. Lab Invest 2009;89(9):1053–62.
87. Hooper ML. The role of the p53 and Rb-1 genes in cancer, development and apoptosis. J Cell Sci Suppl 1994;18:13–7.
88. You H, Mak TW. Crosstalk between p53 and FOXO transcription factors. Cell Cycle 2005;4(1):37–8.
89. Kim YA, Lee WH, Choi TH, et al. Involvement of p21WAF1/CIP1, pRB, Bax and NF-kappaB in induction of growth arrest and apoptosis by resveratrol in human lung carcinoma A549 cells. Int J Oncol 2003;23(4):1143–9.
90. Zhou M, Gu L, Zhu N, et al. Transfection of a dominant-negative mutant NF-kB inhibitor (IkBm) represses p53-dependent apoptosis in acute lymphoblastic leukemia cells: interaction of IkBm and p53. Oncogene 2003;22(50):8137–44.

Frailty and Chronic Diseases in Older Adults

Carlos O. Weiss, MD, MHS

KEYWORDS

• Chronic diseases • Frailty • Epidemiology • Efficiency

THE IMPORTANCE OF FRAILTY AND CHRONIC DISEASES

There are 2 hallmarks of aging that are primary concerns for those trying to improve health for older adults. One is an increased vulnerability to advanced and persistent loss of function that, at least initially, only becomes evident under stress: frailty. Frailty has been described as loss of ability to adapt to stress because of diminished functional reserves.[1,2] According to this simple description, frailty may be said to provide an exaggerated example of how physiologic functions attenuate with aging. The second is the accumulation of pathologic processes that are evident and for which there is substantial agreement about definition: chronic diseases. Frailty and chronic diseases are prime modulators of a person's health trajectory in later life. An understanding of the presence or absence of frailty and chronic diseases constitutes a basic representation of physiologic reserves in old age.

This paper reviews epidemiologic associations among frailty and chronic diseases. Interrelationships among diseases and frailty are discussed, and punished inefficiency is introduced as an explanatory framework for frailty that draws on pathophysiologic relationships caused by chronic diseases and conditions. We use phenotypic definition of frailty as defined in the Cardiovascular Health Studies and in the Women's Health and Aging Studies.[3,4] This definition was chosen because of several considerations. It was one of only 2 attempts to create a standardized and reliable definition using population-based samples of older adults. The other attempt to do this, the cumulative deficit approach by Rockwood[5] and Rockwood and colleagues,[6] is based on a summation of markers of impairment that is inseparable from chronic diseases. Although the cumulative deficit approach is elegant and useful for other purposes, it is not intended to guide a discussion of the mechanisms that cause frailty. We use the prior definition that was created with the purpose of creating a model to facilitate understanding of the physiologic processes that lead to the clinical presentation of

Division of Geriatric Medicine & Gerontology, Johns Hopkins School of Medicine, 5200 Eastern Avenue, Mason F. Lord Center Tower # 707, Baltimore, MD 21224-2734, USA
E-mail address: cweiss9@jhmi.edu

Clin Geriatr Med 27 (2011) 39–52
doi:10.1016/j.cger.2010.08.003
0749-0690/11/$ – see front matter © 2011 Elsevier Inc. All rights reserved.

geriatric.theclinics.com

frailty and to identify therapeutic targets. Such considerations are integral to any discussion of the interface between frailty and chronic diseases. The article by Xue elsewhere in this issue presents a more detailed overview of frailty in later life, and includes discussions of alternative concepts and operational definitions of frailty.

There are several sources of vulnerability in the poor health outcomes that, while being related to frailty, can be considered distinct from intrinsic frailty. How a person interacts with the environment and makes decisions play major roles in modulating the development and course of frailty or diseases. Physiologic frailty may be unobservable outside a specific context made up of environmental features and behavior molded by that environment, and therefore a full measure of frailty would require a matrix comprising physiologic reserves and parameters for interactions with the environment and personal choices. The discussion here focuses on physiologic contributors to changes in function at the individual level and also considers frail individuals with altered physiologic function in the context of interactions with health care systems.

INSIGHTS FROM THE EPIDEMIOLOGY OF FRAILTY AND CHRONIC DISEASES
Epidemiology of Frailty

The prevalence of frailty has been estimated to be 6.9% among older community-dwelling adults in the United States, and it increased within that group from 3.2% among 65- to 70-year-olds to 23.1% among people aged 90 years and older.[3] This prevalence was also higher in women and African Americans[7] or people of Latino origin, although using reference ranges derived from ethnic cohorts may explain some of these differences.[8] Frailty is therefore less prevalent than most chronic diseases that are ranked highly as causes of death or morbidity. The incidence of frailty has been estimated at 71.8/1000 person years in the Cardiovascular Health Study (CHS),[3] 22.5 to 38.7/1000 person years in the Precipitating Events Project,[9] and as high as 191/1000 person years in women from among the one-third most disabled living in the community in the Women's Health and Aging Study I.[10] The onset of frailty may occur most often as weakness, followed by slowness[11]; however, among people who have developed frailty (ie, have at least 3 of the 5 criteria), slowness was found most commonly.[12] The duration of frailty is not long in comparison with most diseases. In 1.5 years, 12.9% to 23.0% of people with frailty recovered to a prefrail state, whereas 13.1% to 20.1% died.[9] Thus, the time spent frail is also less than time spent disabled,[13] because of higher risk of mortality.

Given the prevalence and duration, it follows that a small minority of people who have multimorbidity, several chronic diseases simultaneously, are frail. In CHS, only 9.7% of the older adults with multimorbidity were frail, whereas 67.7% of frail adults had multimorbidity among 9 diseases considered.[3] The mean number of chronic diseases experienced by a frail older adult was roughly 2.1, compared with 1.4 among nonfrail older adults.[7] These findings suggest that frailty is either (1) not caused by mechanisms that are shared with chronic diseases; (2) may be caused by mechanisms that are shared with chronic diseases once the diseases have reached a severe or advanced state; or (3) may be caused by specific interactions between disease-related physiologic impairments that occur less frequently than single diseases, but is unlikely to be caused by 1 or 2 disease pathways alone, except in the case of (2).

Frailty and Chronic Diseases

Table 1 lists the chronic diseases that have been associated with frailty in published cohort studies of older adults that used standardized disease ascertainment.[3,14–16] Starting with the most common chronic disease among the frail, hypertension, the

Table 1
Association of chronic diseases with frailty, in women and overall

| Chronic Disease | Prevalence (%) | | | | Citation(s) |
| | Women | | Overall | | |
	Frail	Nonfrail	Frail	Nonfrail	
Hypertension	60.8	43.4	50.8–53.1	34.0–38.8	1b; 13a; 14b,c
Chronic kidney disease	54.3	42.5	–	–	25b
Osteoarthritis	78.2	48.1	25.9–70.8	9.7–44.8	1b; 13b; 14b
Depressive symptoms	46.3	13.3	–	–	25b
Coronary heart disease	17.2–41.5	5.8–20.8	–	–	12b; 14b
Diabetes mellitus	9.9–21.3	2.6–12.1	13.6–25.0	10.0–12.1	12a; 13; 14b
Chronic lower respiratory tract disease	9.8–15.5	2.5–4.3	12.3–14. 1	7.4–5.8	1b; 12; 13; 14b
Myocardial infarction alone	–	–	8.6–13.3	4.4–7.3	1b; 13
Rheumatoid arthritis	6.4	1.6	–	–	12b
Stroke	4.4	1.1	12.3	3.8	13a; 14b
Peripheral arterial disease	–	–	3.8–14.8	1.5–5.6	1a; 13a
Congestive heart failure	3.5	0.6	12.3–13.6	2.0–3.6	12b; 14b

[a] $P<.05$.
[b] $P<.01$.
[c] Nonfrail group did not include prefrail, sometimes called intermediate group, because prevalence for that group was reported separately. In addition to sample selection, there are differences among cited studies related to disease definition and/or operationalization of frailty criteria that may explain differences. Data for men are not shown because these were not reported in the studies. Chronic lower respiratory tract disease is asthma or chronic obstructive pulmonary disease.

prevalence is shown in descending order among frail and nonfrail older adults to allow absolute and relative comparisons. This comparison is shown for women and overall, because data for men were not reported in the studies that included men. Joint examination of the studies in **Table 1** points to several findings. The prevalence of chronic diseases, even if taken one at a time, is often doubled in older women who are frail, and sometimes increased by a factor of 3 or 4 for less-common diseases for which a tripling or quadrupling is possible. However, there is no single disease-frailty association that seems to be markedly stronger than the rest, even if congestive heart failure and depression are foremost. The nonfrail group did not include the prefrail group, sometimes called intermediate group, in some studies because prevalence for that group was reported separately. In addition, besides sample selection, there were differences related to disease definition and/or operationalization of frailty criteria among cited studies that may have caused small artifacts.

Frailty and Non-Disease Conditions

Some common conditions that are causes or consequences of chronic diseases in older adults have been shown to be associated with frailty. Among these, a poor nutritional state has been strongly implicated by consistent findings that show an increased risk for malnutrition[10] and evidence of low nutrient intake[17–19] in frail older adults. Together with the low activity levels that are part of the frailty definition, these support the hypothesis that energy dysregulation may be a central issue in frailty as it is in congestive heart failure, diabetes, stroke, and chronic lung disease. These diseases were all noted to be associated with frailty in **Table 1**. What has not been determined yet, but is currently being studied, is how frail older adults may experience a redistribution among the compartments that make up total energy expenditure: activity, resting metabolism, thermogenesis related to food intake, and other compartments. In further support of impaired energy throughput as an important pathway in frailty and chronic disease development, anemia has been shown to interact synergistically with cardiovascular disease as a risk factor for frailty with a test for interaction.[14] A review of the many conditions or syndromes that are not conventional diseases but have been hypothesized to shed light on the causes of frailty is outside the scope of this discussion. Notably, inflammation,[20,21] which can be caused by chronic diseases, overlaps with and may lead to a shared contribution to the development of frailty. In addition, frailty has been associated with blood markers of thrombogenicity.[22,23]

Interactions Among Frailty and Chronic Diseases and Conditions and Treatments

Fig. 1 shows how chronic diseases or conditions of varying severity may act alone or in combination, have converging or diverging effects, or lead to the use of therapeutic interventions whose unintended consequences contribute to frailty. As one example, labeled A on the left side of the figure, a person has congestive heart failure, hypothyroidism, and sarcopenia. These chronic diseases and conditions may act through distinct mechanisms that converge to cause an element of frailty if each is mild. In contrast, an example person labeled B on the right side of the figure has severe depression and experiences a more developed frailty phenotype with symptoms and signs that may have a single underlying mechanism but have diverging effects. It is unlikely that any severe chronic disease will affect reserves through just 1 mechanistic pathway or have secondary effects that are restricted to 1 physiologic system. One-to-one correlations between chronic diseases or conditions and frailty are not the rule. Many diseases can converge to cause a single prominent symptom or sign, or a single disease that is severe may cause many diverging symptoms and signs.

This schematic is consistent with the hypothesis that frailty is not disease specific.[4] In addition, the figure illustrates that, when there is access to care, diseases almost always lead to treatments, many of which can have side effects that could contribute to frailty. This possible feed-forward phenomenon among chronic diseases, frailty, and treatment is discussed later. It has been theorized that multimorbidity entails clinically overt diseases, and, distinct from multimorbidity, frailty is an aggregate of subclinical losses of reserve across multiple systems,[24] and may occur in parallel with multimorbidity.[25] These ideas may find some support from research showing that some biologic components of the metabolic syndrome (insulin resistance, inflammation), but not the whole syndrome, predict frailty.[26] Although clinicians caring for

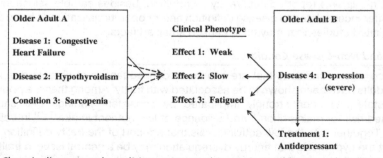

Fig. 1. Chronic diseases and conditions may act alone or in combinations, have converging or diverging effects, or lead to treatments that create frailty.

older adults know of cases in which frailty could never be ascribed to a disease diagnosis, it can be especially challenging to show empirically that frailty that is not disease related.

The possibility of interactions among diseases to cause frailty is a central issue. This possibility has been formally evaluated[27] using methods to test specifically for biologic interactions. In a study of 620 older women, 2 pairs of diseases or conditions were found to have significant biologic interactions that increased the risk of frailty: anemia and depression, and anemia and pulmonary disease. The proportions of the association between the diseases and frailty attributable to an interaction of the 2 diseases were substantial at 56% and 61%, respectively. Smaller interactions may have been detected by a larger study. A similar question has also been studied at the level of continuous physiologic function, rather than binary disease status, with a focus on exercise capacity as the outcome and frailty status as a potential modifier of physiologic reserves.[28] The study examined whether the systems involved in converting energy into lower extremity exercise capacity interact; that is, whether they responded differently to each other, in frail adults, compared with nonfrail, using interactive regression models. The results suggested that key physiologic impairments in lung function, leg strength, and frailty all caused diminished exercise capacity, cumulatively, in disabled older women. Furthermore, and more specifically, the positive effects of pulmonary function on better exercise capacity were significant in the absence of frailty but were muted in frailty, suggesting that integrated functioning could be degraded or uncoupled in frailty. Modulation by frailty status of the cumulative effects of pulmonary function and leg strength on exercise capacity was not statistically significant, possibly because of power limitations imposed by exclusion criteria for exercise testing.

INTERRELATIONSHIPS AMONG FRAILTY AND CHRONIC DISEASES
Empirical Models to Provide Further Support for Theory

The available data derived from the phenotypic approach to frailty support many aspects of the prespecified theory, a benefit and bane of hypothesis-driven research. Frailty meets criteria for a geriatric syndrome because it does not fit within a discrete disease definition category, but is substantially prevalent and involves several organ systems.[12,29] Multidimensionality, or involvement of several physiologic subsystems, is a core characteristic of frailty, such that more than 1 impaired type of function is present.[1,3] However, the data still leave unanswered many questions related to frailty's essential features. The list of physiologic subsystems that should be measured to capture frailty is potentially long,[25,30,31] suggesting that there may be several subtypes of frailty.[32] Unlike many conventional medical disease syndromes, frailty is likely to have multiple potential triggers, or points of entry, some of which correspond closely with advanced chronic disease complicated by malnutrition. As an alternative to the idea that there are subtypes of frailty, it is possible that there are different physiologic states, some dynamic, some suspended, on a frailty pathway. As an example of shifting among physiologic states, frailty may be both a wasting syndrome akin to failure to thrive and coexist with obesity.[33] Similarly, the reduction in heart rate variability recently associated with frailty may have different implications in differing physiologic conditions.[34]

Because of frailty's multidimensionality, attempts to explain its causes are increasingly turning to a nonlinear, complex adaptive systems modeling approach that can provide new analyses of the relationship between frailty and chronic diseases. There has been a call to measure dynamics in response to a stressor,[2] making sure to compare frail and nonfrail individuals responding to the same stressor. Such research should provide critical information because responses to stress engage feedback loops involving more than 1 physiologic system, some of which will be impaired in older adults with chronic diseases. These feedback loops may behave differently because of setpoint alterations caused by disease or the level of stressful stimulus. In such a system, small differences in starting levels can lead to divergent outcomes because a small stressor can be either diminished or magnified. Frailty is therefore an emergent property in a complex nonlinear system.[35] The important components are the dynamics, not just the individual functions, so interdependent risk factors and nonlinearity are expected. Instead of searching for mechanisms by holding everything except 1 variable constant, in a traditional experimental mindset, in the case of frailty it is expected that studying specific elements in isolation or one at a time cannot lead to a true understanding of the system, just as studying different cars and drivers in isolation cannot lead to a prediction of when or where traffic jams will occur.

To identify therapeutic targets in a complex dynamic system like frailty, it is necessary to distinguish compensatory mechanisms from primary derangements caused by disease. This distinction is particularly important because frailty may emerge when several diseased physiologic subsystems begin to operate semiautonomously. A strategy that is optimal for a physiologic subsystem (eg, preservation of the kidney's ability to filtrate) may have effects that are not optimal for the organism (eg, an increase in systemic vascular resistance and left ventricular end-diastolic pressure).[36] This example is discussed later. The uncoupling of benefit to the whole organism from compensatory strategies that, in isolation, provide benefits on a smaller scale provides refinement for the general hypothesis that frailty is the result of impaired homeostasis in several systems.

Punished Inefficiency as a Conceptual Framework for Frailty and Chronic Disease

Based on a complex dynamic systems approach, attention to the central importance of fatigue and exhaustion for frailty, and an understanding of physiologic costs and gains, punished inefficiency proposes that having several physiologic impairments leads not simply to loss of ability and proportional disadvantages but to physiologic inefficiencies. These inefficiencies may become manifest as frailty, often in the presence of disease. As a consequence, frail older adults may perform less external work to avoid spending more out of a smaller pool of internal resources. Stress imposed on frail older adults can strengthen this negative feedback on activity, and lead to disuse and to worsening of chronic disease states.[37]

Impaired of energy flow has been recognized as a prime candidate for changes caused by aging. Physiologic functioning is counterentropic because it provides a stimulus that sustains supporting physiologic structures through healthy feedback.[38] Conversely, age-associated blunted or reduced physiologic function leads to a loss of supporting physiologic structures, and even a restructuring of homeostasis.[39] This theory has been hypothesized to also apply to changes that occur because of chronic diseases, leading to frailty.[32]

Punished inefficiency proposes, first, that energy should not be studied as a rate using time as the denominator, as is most commonly done in an energy expenditure approach (eg, mL O_2/kg/time elapsed). Energy flow should also be measured as a rate using work achieved as a denominator, an energy efficiency approach, sometimes also referred to as energy economy or energy cost (eg, mL O_2/kg/m traveled). Usual or preferred gait speed, a frailty criterion, provides an example of how energy efficiency provides critical guidance. Among frailty criteria, slowed gait speed is the strongest predictor of functional dependence or disability.[40–42] It is now believed that the energy efficiency of walking explains preferred walking speed. The brain selects the most energy efficient speed as its preferred speed, also identifiable as the nadir in a curve expressing the relationships between energy costs on the y-axis and gait speed on the x-axis.[43–45] This relationship illustrates that reduced function, an obvious consequence of physiologic impairments, may not be as important as inefficiency for identifying the optimal physiologic setpoint for an individual. Reduced function on an external and nonbiologic per-unit-time scale may not provide information that leads to an understanding of how homeostatic relationships were reorganized.

Frail older adults with impairments, compared with nonfrail older adults, can consume more energy to achieve normal levels of work, and thereby slow down to both normalize energy expenditure and, perhaps more importantly, perform tasks with as little loss of efficiency as possible. Although, to a casual observer, it may appear to be doing less, walking with physiologic impairments is inefficient, as anyone who has tried to walk up stairs with an injured leg or foot can attest. In addition, because disease-related pathologies create a smaller pool of available energy, behavior is affected by conditions of scarcity. In this way, it may be possible to better explain the behavior of frail individuals. They walk more slowly, arrive at their destination later, and use more energy to cover the same distance.

The implications of this theory, if it is further validated, are that frailty comprises a synergistic interaction whereby individuals with loss of reserves also experience loss of efficiency in a manner that is detrimental to maintaining adequate physiologic function. Many physiologic relationships are consistent with this idea. For example, the heart muscle performs more work (cardiac output, on a conventional per-unit-time basis) as end-diastolic pressure in the left ventricle increases. However, physiologic impairments related to heart failure lead to the well-known shift off the Frank-Starling curve, whereby muscle fibers are no longer at optimal length. Increased demand on the heart muscle is not translated as efficiently into increased cardiac output. The amount of oxygen consumed to achieve the same amount of oxygen delivery is increased. In a possible example of homeostatic rearrangement, there are data to suggest that adaptation in this manner can even fail to occur in older adults, which constitutes a further worsening of efficiency than a shift in the curve.[46] Loss of efficiency is a general phenomenon, because physiologic impairments in exercise capacity lead to an increase in the number of muscle fibers that need to be recruited to create the same amount of force. These changes result in recruitment of larger muscle units that are more susceptible to fatigue.[47] Research using an efficiency model, such as usual gait speed[48,49] or the oxygen uptake efficiency slope that examines the milliliters of oxygen taken up per volume of air moved through the lungs,[50] has identified elegant predictors of physiologic reserve. **Fig. 2** provides a general form for studying physiologic function through the use of an efficiency index comprising units of cost (eg, oxygen consumed) per amount gained (eg, meters traveled, ions transported). Studying changes in efficiency should provide a way to assess when a compensatory strategy improves function. This assessment is especially important in frail older adults with diseases because of the potential for opposing effects from similar responses whose physiologic context is incompletely understood.[51] In addition, although it has been suspected that many geriatric syndromes are self-sustaining,[29] physiologic inefficiency, especially if it is punished, provides a framework for specifying testable hypotheses related to physiologic changes associated with diseases and aging.

Reduced efficiency may often be confronted uncharitably by conditions of increased external demand, or *punished*, creating a feedback loop that further

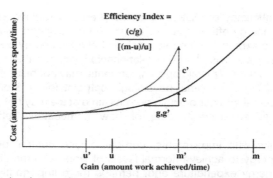

Fig. 2. Efficiency index that can be used to understand loss of optimization in frailty. Physiologic function can be studied in terms of efficiency, not simply expenditure over time. The units of this efficiency index are resource spent/work gained. c, cost in response to stimulus to increase function; g, gain in response to stimulus to increase function; M, function at maximum; u, usual function. The m, u, g, c, and solid line correspond with the healthy state. In the frail state identified by prime variables and the dotted line, maximum function is lowered (m−m′); usual function is lowered to a lesser degree (u−u′) to maintain similar physiologic expenditures on the y-axis; proportional function [(m′−u′)/u′] can be preserved; and more resources are spent to achieve the same gain, that is, the cost slope is greater (c′/g′>c/g).

promotes inefficiency. Most older adults with a major chronic disease have at least 2 of them.[52] Many physiologic examples of inefficiency are available for an older adult with at least 2 chronic diseases, and expanding the scope of investigation from physiology to behaviors and treatments will further exemplify this phenomenon.

However, even though most frail older adults have, and receive treatments for, chronic diseases, the effects of care received from a system that was not designed for the frail have received little attention in frailty research. An incomplete or distorted understanding of frailty on the part of health care providers can lead to perverse responses, whereby the level of demands placed on a person by the health care system are inversely proportional to physiologic reserves. **Table 2** presents a construct of how frail older adults with chronic diseases experience more formal care stressors, contributing to punished inefficiency. In conditions of low physiologic reserve (as can be expected in individuals with several chronic diseases), increased demands can dissipate limited resources and lead to an amplification of physiologic inefficiency. **Fig. 3**A, B illustrate this phenomenon in older adults in the National Health and Nutrition Examination Survey (1999–2001), a sample representing community-dwelling people. Hospitalization rates in **Fig. 3**A, and number of prescribed medications in **Fig. 3**B, increase synergistically according to one criterion of frailty (slower usual gait speed) and the presence of chronic diseases. In the real-world context of receiving health care, frailty can have a feed-forward negative effect on activity.[53]

The motivation for understanding punished inefficiency is to reverse frailty, possibly by improving energy efficiency in older individuals through appropriate therapies that augment compensatory strategies. As an example, resistance training holds the potential to improve efficiency during real-life activities in older adults.[54] It is imperative to target treatment among frail older adults because a treatment can be administered in the wrong physiologic context can contribute to a rearrangement of interactions among physiologic systems that is harmful. In good health, such, a rearrangement of processes is unlikely for complex, highly redundant physiologic processes, with are exceptions where there is a crucial gate mechanism, such as cardiac pacemaking.[55] In contrast, some physiologic processes and many behaviors

Table 2
How frail older adults with chronic diseases experience more formal care stressors, causing punished inefficiency

Individual Health Status	Involvement with Formal Health Care	Combined Result
In frail with chronic diseases, the intrinsic physiologic reserves listed are decreased	In frail with chronic diseases, the extrinsic stressors imposed by disease care are increased	Intrinsic resilience and extrinsic stressors are related inversely through bidirectional feedback
Structural Changes (Examples)		
Communication (rods and cones in eyes, hair cells in ears, nerve cells)	Number of people providing care (primary care, subspecialists, mental health)	Decreased ability to receive an increased amount and variety of sensory input
Dimensionality across scales (loglinear hormonal relationships)	Number and type of visits (urgent, follow-up)	
Coupling connections across systems (nutrient availability, oxygen use and thermogenesis)	Number and type of tests and interventions (diagnostic procedures)	
Functional Changes (Examples)		
Range of stimulus that can be processed (levels of light, sound waves)	Emergency care (emergency room, hospital)	Decreased ability to reconcile and create targeted response to an increased amount and variety of stressors
Dynamic range of function (tendon elasticity, renal clearance, gas ventilation, blood oxygen carrying capacity, mental multitasking)	Duration of illness episodes (deconditioning)	
Dimensionality (maintenance of muscle mass, salt and water balance, life space)	Locations of care and health care information	
Ability to qualitatively change processing (speed up, walk on different surfaces, efficiency)	Iatrogenic complications and conflicting therapies (nosocomial infections, delirium, deep vein thrombosis)	
Anatomic integrity (ulcerations, tooth loss, amputations)	Reversals of improving trajectory (exacerbations of coexisting conditions)	
Emergent Manifestations (Examples)		
Impairments are synonymous with diminished adaptive capacity (falls causing injuries)	Increased use and spending	Diminished therapeutic effectiveness, and increased disability and death
Integrative ability is also impaired leading to energetic inefficiency (early fatigue)		

Formal health care refers to paid activities that an older adult would not do if they were healthy. Informal health care by unpaid caregivers is important and not illustrated here because of space constraints.

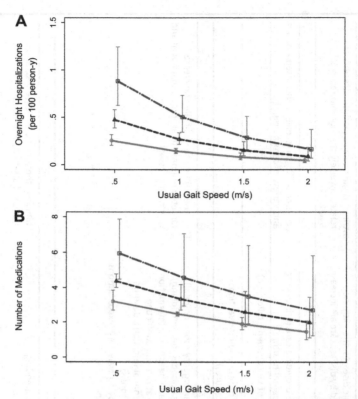

Fig. 3. (*A*) Rate of overnight hospitalization among older adults in NHANES 1999 to 2002, according to usual gait speed and presence of 1, 3, or 5 chronic diseases. (*B*) Number of medications taken by older adults in NHANES 1999 to 2002, according to usual gait speed and presence of 1, 3, or 5 chronic diseases. Circle/solid orange line, 1 chronic disease; triangle/dashed blue line, 3 chronic diseases; square/dot-dashed red line, 5 chronic diseases. Bars are 95% confidence intervals. Data are from people aged 65 years and older in NHANES 1999 to 2002 (n = 3953) and estimates are from multivariable negative binomial regression models using survey weights. Gait speed and chronic diseases were significant predictors of both outcomes (*P*<.01) and for number of medications an interaction term was also significant (*P* = .003). Residual age difference was not a significant contributor after adjustment for gait speed and chronic diseases and was removed from final models.

by frail people with chronic diseases are highly reflexive (ie, dependent on sensory input for deciding the type of response) and therefore more capable of shifts or reversals that short-circuit homeostatic mechanisms, resulting in a negative feed-forward effect. For this reason, future work on the interactions of frail older adults with the health care system appears to be highly important.

DO INTERVENTIONS THAT PREVENT OR TREAT CHRONIC DISEASES ALSO PREVENT FRAILTY?

The current standard is to treat geriatric syndromes, even when incomplete understanding complicates diagnosis and management must be directed at manifestations, not underlying causes.[29] However, caution seems warranted before approaching frailty this way because it is possible that there are physiologic subtypes of frailty, and response to an intervention is likely to vary according to several factors, such as the level of functioning of several interdependent physiologic systems. Given current understanding, there is a limited basis for directly treating frailty. Exercise has been shown to have the potential to reverse several non–disease-specific characteristics of frailty.[56,57] An important opportunity to improve current understanding of the causes of frailty would arise if frailty were measured as an outcome in randomized controlled trials of disease-based therapies. For example, observational data currently do not support the idea that use of statins, with their pleiotropic effects on lipid levels and inflammation, lowers incidence of frailty.[58] However, data from randomized trials are needed to gain a clearer understanding of whether statins, or other pharmacologic therapies, have a biologic effect on the development or prognosis of frailty. The major barrier to gaining such an understanding from randomized trials is a failure to measure frailty as an outcome in large trials of older adults.[30,59] In particular, frailty holds promise as a treatment effect modifier that identifies a small but vulnerable subset in whom treatment can be more or less efficacious.[57]

SUMMARY

The goal of geriatric medicine is to continually improve how older adults can avoid or be affected by the diseases and frailty that often accompany later life. Although it only affects a minority of older adults, frailty is highly predictive of adverse health outcomes. The associations between frailty and chronic diseases can inform a next generation of models to understand frailty as an emergent property in a complex adaptive system. Punished inefficiency may serve as one of these models to distinguish physiologic compensations from impairments and avoid feedback loops that cause or accelerate frailty. The effects on frailty of treatment directed at chronic diseases have received little attention thus far.

REFERENCES

1. Fried LP, Xue QL, Cappola AR, et al. Nonlinear multisystem physiological dysregulation associated with frailty in older women: implications for etiology and treatment. J Gerontol A Biol Sci Med Sci 2009;64:1049–57.
2. Varadhan R, Seplaki CL, Xue QL, et al. Stimulus-response paradigm for characterizing the loss of resilience in homeostatic regulation associated with frailty. Mech Ageing Dev 2008;129(11):666–70.
3. Fried LP, Tangen CM, Walston J, et al. Frailty in older adults: evidence for a phenotype. J Gerontol A Biol Sci Med Sci 2001;56(3):M146–56.
4. Fried LP, Walston J. Frailty and failure to thrive. In: Hazzard WR, Blass JP, Halter JB, et al, editors. Principles of geriatric medicine and gerontology. New York: McGraw-Hill; 2003. p. 1487–502.
5. Rockwood K. What would make a definition of frailty successful? Age Ageing 2005;34(5):432–4.
6. Rockwood K, Mogilner A, Mitnitski A. Changes with age in the distribution of a frailty index. Mech Ageing Dev 2004;125(7):517–9.
7. Hirsch C, Anderson ML, Newman A, et al. The association of race with frailty: the Cardiovascular Health Study. Ann Epidemiol 2006;16:545–53.
8. Espinoza SE, Hazuda HP. Frailty in older Mexican-American and European-American adults: is there an ethnic disparity? J Am Geriatr Soc 2008;56:1744–9.
9. Gill TM. Transitions between frailty states among community-living older persons. Arch Intern Med 2006;166:418–23.

10. Semba RD, Blaum CS, Bartali B, et al. Denture use, malnutrition, frailty, and mortality among older women living in the community. J Nutr Health Aging 2006;10(2):161-7.
11. Xue QL, Bandeen-Roche K, Varadhan R, et al. Initial manifestations of frailty criteria and the development of frailty phenotype in the Women's Health and Aging Study II. J Gerontol A Biol Sci Med Sci 2008;63(9):984-90.
12. Bandeen-Roche K, Xue QL, Ferrucci L, et al. Phenotype of frailty: characterization in the women's health and aging studies. J Gerontol A Biol Sci Med Sci 2006; 61(3):262-6.
13. Thorpe RJ Jr, Weiss C, Xue QL, et al. Transitions among disability levels or death in African American and white older women. J Gerontol A Biol Sci Med Sci 2009; 64(6):670-4.
14. Chaves PH, Semba RD, Leng SX, et al. Impact of anemia and cardiovascular disease on frailty status of community-dwelling older women: the Women's Health and Aging Studies I and II. J Gerontol A Biol Sci Med Sci 2005;60(6):729-35.
15. Cesari M, Leeuwenburgh C, Lauretani F, et al. Frailty syndrome and skeletal muscle: results from the Invecchiare in Chianti study. Am J Clin Nutr 2006; 83(5):1142-8.
16. Woods NF, LaCroix AZ, Gray SL, et al. Frailty: emergence and consequences in women aged 65 and older in the Women's Health Initiative Observational Study. J Am Geriatr Soc 2005;53(8):1321-30.
17. Bartali B, Frongillo EA, Bandinelli S, et al. Low nutrient intake is an essential component of frailty in older persons. J Gerontol A Biol Sci Med Sci 2006; 61(6):589-93.
18. Michelon E, Blaum C, Semba RD, et al. Vitamin and carotenoid status in older women: associations with the frailty syndrome. J Gerontol A Biol Sci Med Sci 2006;61(6):600-7.
19. Semba RD, Bartali B, Zhou J, et al. Low serum micronutrient concentrations predict frailty among older women living in the community. J Gerontol A Biol Sci Med Sci 2006;61(6):594-9.
20. Leng SX, Xue QL, Tian J, et al. Inflammation and frailty in older women. J Am Geriatr Soc 2007;55(6):864-71.
21. Schmaltz HN, Fried LP, Xue QL, et al. Chronic cytomegalovirus infection and inflammation are associated with prevalent frailty in community-dwelling older women. J Am Geriatr Soc 2005;53(5):747-54.
22. Walston J, McBurnie MA, Newman A, et al. Frailty and activation of the inflammation and coagulation systems with and without clinical comorbidities: results from the Cardiovascular Health Study. Arch Intern Med 2002;162(20):2333-41.
23. Folsom AR, Boland LL, Cushman M, et al. Frailty and risk of venous thromboembolism in older adults. J Gerontol A Biol Sci Med Sci 2007;62(1):79-82.
24. Fried LP, Ferrucci L, Darer J, et al. Untangling the concepts of disability, frailty, and comorbidity: implications for improved targeting and care. J Gerontol A Biol Sci Med Sci 2004;59(3):255-63.
25. Ferrucci L, Windham BG, Fried L. Frailty in older persons. Genus LXI 2005;1: 39-53.
26. Barzilay JI, Blaum C, Moore T, et al. Insulin resistance and inflammation as precursors of frailty: the Cardiovascular Health Study. Arch Intern Med 2007; 167(7):635-41.
27. Chang SS, Weiss CO, Xue Q, et al. Patterns of comorbid inflammatory diseases in frail older women: the Women's Health and Aging Studies I and II. J Gerontol A Biol Sci Med Sci 2010;65:407-13.

28. Weiss CO, Hoenig HH, Varadhan R, et al. Relationships of cardiac, pulmonary, and muscle reserves and frailty to exercise capacity in older women. J Gerontol A Biol Sci Med Sci 2010;65:287–94.

29. Inouye SK, Studenski S, Tinetti ME, et al. Geriatric syndromes: clinical, research, and policy implications of a core geriatric concept. J Am Geriatr Soc 2007;55(5): 780–91.

30. Ferrucci L, Guralnik J, Studenski S, et al. Designing randomized, controlled trials aimed at preventing or delaying functional decline and disability in frail, older persons: a consensus report. J Am Geriatr Soc 2004;52(4):625–34.

31. Hamerman D. Toward an understanding of frailty. Ann Intern Med 1999;130(11): 945–50.

32. Fried LP, Hadley EC, Walston JD, et al. From bedside to bench: research agenda for frailty. Sci Aging Knowledge Environ 2005;2005(31):pe24.

33. Blaum CS, Xue QL, Michelon E, et al. The association between obesity and the frailty syndrome in older women: the Women's Health and Aging Studies. J Am Geriatr Soc 2005;53(6):927–34.

34. Chaves P, Varadhan R, Lipsitz LA, et al. Physiological complexity underlying heart rate dynamics and frailty status in community-dwelling older women. J Am Geriatr Soc 2008;56(9):1698–703.

35. Seely AJ, Christou NV. Multiple organ dysfunction syndrome: exploring the paradigm of complex nonlinear systems. Crit Care Med 2000;28(7):2193–200.

36. Youn H, Gastner MT, Jeong H. Price of anarchy in transportation networks: efficiency and optimality control. Phys Rev Lett 2008;101(12):128701.

37. Bortz WM 2nd. Aging as entropy. Exp Gerontol 1986;21(4–5):321–8.

38. Bortz WM 2nd. The physics of frailty. J Am Geriatr Soc 1993;41(9):1004–8.

39. Bortz WM 2nd. A conceptual framework of frailty: a review. J Gerontol A Biol Sci Med Sci 2002;57(5):M283–8.

40. Boyd CM, Xue QL, Simpson CF, et al. Frailty, hospitalization, and progression of disability in a cohort of disabled older women. Am J Med 2005;118(11): 1225–31.

41. Purser JL, Weinberger M, Cohen HJ, et al. Walking speed predicts health status and hospital costs for frail elderly male veterans. J Rehabil Res Dev 2005;42(4): 535–46.

42. Rothman MD, Leo-Summers L, Gill TM. Prognostic significance of potential frailty criteria. J Am Geriatr Soc 2008;56(12):2211–6.

43. Willis WT, Ganley KJ, Herman RM. Fuel oxidation during human walking. Metabolism 2005;54(6):793–9.

44. Holt KG, Hamill J, Andres RO. Predicting the minimal energy costs of human walking. Med Sci Sports Exerc 1991;23(4):491–8.

45. Holt KJ, Jeng SF, Rr RR, et al. Energetic cost and stability during human walking at the preferred stride velocity. J Mot Behav 1995;27(2):164–78.

46. Pendergast DR, Fisher NM, Calkins E. Cardiovascular, neuromuscular, and metabolic alterations with age leading to frailty. J Gerontol 1993;48(Spec No):61–7.

47. Edgerton VR, Roy RR, Allen DL, et al. Adaptations in skeletal muscle disuse or decreased-use atrophy. Am J Phys Med Rehabil 2002;81(Suppl 11):S127–47.

48. Studenski S, Perera S, Wallace D, et al. Physical performance measures in the clinical setting. J Am Geriatr Soc 2003;51(3):314–22.

49. Guralnik JM, Ferrucci L, Pieper CF, et al. Lower extremity function and subsequent disability: consistency across studies, predictive models, and value of gait speed alone compared with the short physical performance battery. J Gerontol A Biol Sci Med Sci 2000;55(4):M221–31.

50. Hollenberg M, Tager IB. Oxygen uptake efficiency slope: an index of exercise performance and cardiopulmonary reserve requiring only submaximal exercise. J Am Coll Cardiol 2000;36(1):194–201.
51. Weiss CO, Hoenig HM, Fried LP. Compensatory strategies used by older adults facing mobility disability. Arch Phys Med Rehabil 2007;88(9):1217–20.
52. Weiss CO, Boyd CM, Yu Q, et al. Patterns of prevalent major chronic disease among older adults in the United States. JAMA 2007;298(10):1160–2.
53. Xue QL, Fried LP, Glass TA, et al. Life-Space constriction, development of frailty, and the competing risk of mortality: the Women's Health and Aging Study I. Am J Epidemiol 2008;167:240–8.
54. Hartman MJ, Fields DA, Byrne NM, et al. Resistance training improves metabolic economy during functional tasks in older adults. J Strength Cond Res 2007;21(1): 91–5.
55. Greenstein JL, Hinch R, Winslow RL. Mechanisms of excitation-contraction coupling in an integrative model of the cardiac ventricular myocyte. Biophys J 2006;90(1):77–91.
56. Fiatarone MA, O'Neill EF, Ryan ND, et al. Exercise training and nutritional supplementation for physical frailty in very elderly people. N Engl J Med 1994;330(25): 1769–75.
57. Faber MJ, Bosscher RJ, Chin APMJ, et al. Effects of exercise programs on falls and mobility in frail and pre-frail older adults: a multicenter randomized controlled trial. Arch Phys Med Rehabil 2006;87(7):885–96.
58. LaCroix AZ, Gray SL, Aragaki A, et al. Statin use and incident frailty in women aged 65 years or older: prospective findings from the Women's Health Initiative Observational Study. J Gerontol A Biol Sci Med Sci 2008;63(4):369–75.
59. Bhasin S, Cress E, Espeland MA, et al. Functional outcomes for clinical trials in frail older persons: time to be moving. J Gerontol A Biol Sci Med Sci 2008; 63(2):160–4.

The Frail Renin-Angiotensin System

Peter M. Abadir, MD

KEYWORDS

- Renin-angiotensin system • Cardiovascular disease
- Apoptosis • AT1R • Oxidative stress • AT2R • Inflammation

THE RENIN-ANGIOTENSIN SYSTEM

The renin-angiotensin system (RAS) is a hormonal system that is of vital importance not only in the regulation of arterial blood pressure and salt balance, but also in many physiologic and pathophysiologic mechanisms in almost every organ system.[1–3] The system consists mainly of a 2-step enzymatic cascade catalyzed by renin and angiotensin-converting enzyme (ACE), generating angiotensin II (Ang II), a single bioactive peptide. Ang II, the main RAS effector hormone, acts through 2 receptor subtypes, Ang II types 1 and 2 receptors (AT1R and AT2R) (**Fig. 1**).[4,5] Both the receptor types belong to the G protein–coupled receptor family but differ in terms of tissue distribution and cell signaling pathways. Most of the functions of Ang II are carried through AT1R. The role and biologic functions of AT2R are less studied. It has been documented that AT2R inhibits and antagonizes AT1R-mediated functions,[6–9] and when stimulated by Ang II, AT2R exerts effects that are the opposite of AT1R, including antiinflammatory,[10] antiproliferative,[10] and antiapoptotic actions (**Table 1**).[11] Hence, AT2R may play an important role in vascular aging.

Evidence suggests that virtually every organ system in the human body possesses a local RAS. The components of RAS are present in peripheral tissues such as vasculature, kidneys, adrenal glands, heart, and immune cells, all of which locally produce Ang II.[12–14] These local systems seem to be independently regulated and compartmentalized from the plasma circulation.[15]

Binding of Ang II to AT1R or AT2R activates various complex signal transduction pathways. Through AT1R, Ang II activates various intracellular protein kinases. These intracellular signaling cascades include receptor- and non-receptor–mediated tyrosine kinases, serine/threonine kinases, mitogen-activated protein kinase (MAPK) family (extracellular signal-regulated kinase, c-Jun N terminal kinase, and p38MAPK), p70 S6 kinase, Akt/PKB (protein kinase B), and various protein kinase C isoforms.[16–19] These intracellular signals have been linked to vascular remodeling through induction of hypertrophy, hyperplasia, and migration of vascular smooth muscle cells.[16–19] In contrast, AT2R signals through 3 major transduction pathways

Division of Geriatric Medicine and Gerontology, Johns Hopkins University School of Medicine, John R. Burton Pavilion, 5505 Hopkins Bayview Circle, Baltimore, MD 21224, USA
E-mail address: pabadir1@jhmi.edu

Clin Geriatr Med 27 (2011) 53–65
doi:10.1016/j.cger.2010.08.004
0749-0690/11/$ – see front matter © 2011 Elsevier Inc. All rights reserved.

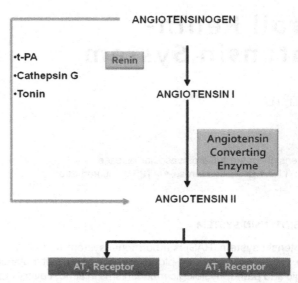

Fig. 1. The steps in the biochemical pathway that is involved in the formation of the most biologically potent angiotensin peptide Ang II and its interaction with angiotensin receptors. The enzymes renin converts angiotensinogen to angiotensin I, which in turn is converted via angiotensin converting enzyme to Angiotensin II. Other enzymes that facilitate alternative pathways for the formation of Ang II are tPA, cathepsin G, and tonin. tPA, tissue plasminogen activator.

that seem to oppose the actions of AT1R: (1) activation of various protein phosphatases causing protein dephosphorylation, (2) activation of the nitric oxide/cyclic GMP system, and (3) stimulation of phospholipase A_2, with subsequent release of arachidonic acid.[20] Of these pathways, MAPK and phosphotyrosine phosphatase (PTP) have been the most studied classic signaling cascade of AT1R and AT2R.[21–25] AT1R activates MAPK cascade, whereas AT2R inhibits MAPK and activates PTP.[24] The influence of cross talk between AT1R and AT2R on activation of these signaling pathways is still largely unknown.

CHANGES IN RAS WITH AGING

Most of the studies on the effect of aging on RAS have been done in animal models. The effects of aging on RAS have been studied in tissues and in circulation. There

Table 1
Opposing functions of AT1R and AT2R, which might be linked to aging

AT1R	AT2R
Vasoconstriction	Vasodilatation
Cell growth	Antigrowth
Cell proliferation	Cell differentiation
Antinatriuresis	Natriuresis
Production of O_2^-	Production of nitric oxide
Stimulation of fibroblast proliferation and collagen synthesis	Inhibition of fibroblast proliferation
Apoptosis	Antiapoptosis

seems to be a differential regulation of the circulating and intrarenal RAS during aging.[26] On the tissue-specific level, renal Ang II content increases in older animals.[27] In contrast, aging is associated with a decline in the concentration of the components of the circulating RAS in animals, including reduction in renal tissue renin messenger RNA levels, juxtaglomerular cell renin content, responsiveness of renin release to various challenges, and plasma renin and Ang II levels.[27–33] The decline in the concentration of the components of the circulating RAS during aging may be a consequence of the age-related increase in pressure, because plasma Ang II levels do not decline in rats without increased pressure during aging.[26] The reduction in the levels of the circulating RAS components may also have predisposed to the increased renal vasoconstrictor responses to exogenously administered Ang II in older animals.[27] Upregulation of AT1R has been observed in both the heart and the vasculature,[1,2] suggesting an important role of RAS in senescence. On the other hand, AT2R is expressed in large quantities in fetal tissues but its expression decreases in the neonatal period and reaches a comparatively low level in the adult animal.[34] However, the capacity for AT2R reexpression is retained in the adult, because upregulation is a common response to circumstances of cardiovascular tissue damage, such as myocardial infarction, heart failure, and hypertension.[27,35–37] The only available studies on microvascular AT2R expression and action in humans demonstrate that AT2R expression can be induced chronically in hypertensive diabetic subjects by AT1R blockade and, under these circumstances, mediates vasodilation.[27,37] However, the interpretation of these studies and their applicability in human studies is still an area of debate.

There is evidence that an altered ratio between AT1R and AT2R levels may result in elevated blood pressure and induction of inflammation.[38] The contribution of changes in the expression of AT1R and AT2R to the increased production of inflammatory cytokines observed in older individuals is yet to be explored. It also seems that the use of AT1R blockade increases AT2R activity in vivo.[39,40] Beneficial actions of AT1R blockers on remodeling and cardiac fibrosis were completely abolished by simultaneous AT2R blockade, suggesting that such beneficial effects are because of AT2R activation rather than AT1R blockade.[41–43]

How aging might influence RAS is still largely unknown. Genetic and environmental factors may contribute[44] but fail to account entirely for any changes with age. There is evidence from human monozygotic twin studies that methylation patterns can change with aging.[45] The process of aging and development is accompanied by selective methylation of genes that are not needed for function of the differentiated cell. Evidence from animal and human studies suggests that in utero expression of the angiotensin receptors is regulated by methylation of the angiotensin receptor genes.[46,47] However, no studies are available on the effect of aging on the regulation of AT1R and AT2R and their genes in humans. Given the importance of these receptors in performing the major functions of RAS and the gap in knowledge related to how aging triggers and affects these systems, studies as proposed here may have important implications for human health.

RAS AND ITS ROLE IN CHRONIC INFLAMMATION AND FRAILTY IN OLDER ADULTS

Inappropriate, chronic, low-grade inflammation is implicated in the pathogenesis of many common and disabling diseases in older adults. Most of these diseases are slowly progressive and have a clear association with advancing age.[48–50] In addition, chronic inflammation is associated with functional decline, frailty, and increased mortality.[51,52] The clinical criteria for frailty include weight loss, low levels of activity, muscle weakness, exhaustion, and slow walking speed.[51]

The causes that trigger chronic inflammatory activation in older adults are likely heterogeneous and include multiple chronic disease states, redox imbalance, senescent cells, and increased body fat.[53–57] These triggers act through nuclear factor κB signal transduction, which leads to increased expression of multiple inflammatory mediators including tumor necrosis factor (TNF) α, interleukin (IL) 1b, IL-6, cyclooxygenase 2, and inducible nitric oxide synthase.[53–55] The inflammatory cytokine IL-6, total white blood cells, neutrophils, and monocytes have also been identified as significant correlates of frailty in older populations.[58,59] Although the cause cannot be proven from these studies, the consistent and reproducible associations between increased expression of markers of inflammation and frailty in older adults suggest that inflammatory pathways are more active in frail older adults than in nonfrail adults and that chronic inflammation worsens disease status, leading to muscle strength decline and stem cell failure.[48,60] Hence, chronic inflammation may play an important role in late life decline. Frailty status provides an important in vivo model for chronic inflammation and etiology of inflammation and for RAS change.

Substantial evidence confirms the role of RAS in activation of inflammatory pathways. Most of the functions of Ang II are carried through AT1R. The role and biologic functions of AT2R are less studied. It has been reported that AT2R inhibits and antagonizes AT1R-mediated functions (see **Table 1**).[6–9] The activation of AT1R has a powerful proinflammatory effect.[61] AT1R actions include induction of reactive oxygen species,[62] hypertrophy and apoptosis,[11] and stimulation of fibroblast proliferation and collagen synthesis.[63] AT1R antagonists exert cardiovascular protection, in part through their vascular antiinflammatory effects.[64] AT1R activation affects cytokine levels by increasing IL-6,[65] TNF-α,[66–70] and interferon gamma production[71] and decreasing nitric oxide and cyclic GMP production.[72] AT1R expression seems to be limiting for the effect of Ang II. Upregulation of AT1R expression enhances the action of Ang II in vitro as well as in vivo.[73]

The molecular mechanisms through which angiotensin receptors manipulate cytokines production and chronic inflammation remain unclear (**Fig. 2**). Ang II activates the signal transducer and activator of transcription proteins 3 (STAT3).[74] STAT3 is a key signal transduction protein that mediates cell differentiation, proliferation, apoptosis, inflammation, and tumor cell evasion of the immune system.[75] Binding sites have been identified for STAT3 within the promoter region of TNF-α.[76] Mutation of the 3 base pairs of the STAT3 binding site had considerable effects on the promoter activity, demonstrating that STAT3 upregulates TNF-α expression.[76]

To date, few have studies examined the influence of increased inflammation on RAS. In animal models IL-6, released locally, contributes substantially to the vascular dysfunction produced by Ang II.[77] Treatment of mice with IL-6 for 18 days increased vascular AT1R expression.[78] Because the upregulation of AT1R expression in vitro and in vivo is involved in IL-6–induced propagation of oxidative stress and endothelial dysfunction, the interaction of the proinflammatory cytokine IL-6 with RAS may represent an important pathogenetic mechanism in inflammatory diseases in older population.

AGING RAS—DISEASE INTERACTIONS CULMINATING IN THE DEVELOPMENT OF FRAILTY

RAS contributes to the pathogenesis of several human diseases that have a clear association with advanced aging, including hypertension, myocardial infarction, congestive heart failure, stroke, atrial fibrillation, coronary artery disease, diabetes, and nephropathy. Large population studies have clearly demonstrated that both

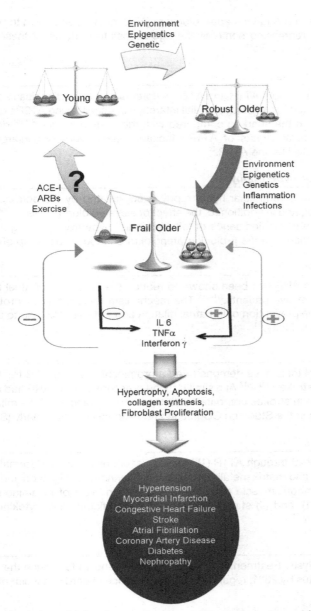

Fig. 2. A hypothetical model for changes in the angiotensin receptors with aging and/or frailty, resulting in increased production of cytokines, pathologic changes, and development/worsening of diseases. Note that with robust aging, the balance is maintained between the angiotensin receptors despite decrease in both AT1R (*circles in right pan*) and AT2R (*circles in left pan*). With development of frailty that balance is tipped toward more expression of AT1R and less AT2R predisposing to increased cytokine production, which further widens the gap by increasing the expression of AT1R and reducing expression of AT2R. ACEi, ACE inhibitor; ARBs, Ang II receptor blockers.

ACE inhibitors and Ang II receptor blockers (ARB) have been shown to be effective in preventing or regressing some of the age-associated effects of these diseases in humans and animals.[79–81]

Myocardial Infarction

The expression of both AT1R and AT2R is upregulated in cardiac tissue after myocardial infarction. Induction of myocardial infarction in mice lacking AT2Rs caused significant damage to the heart as compared with the wild-type mice,[42,82] demonstrating that the beneficial effects of AT1R blockade after myocardial infarction may be partially mediated by the AT2R.[83]

Left Ventricular Hypertrophy

The extent of left ventricular hypertrophy is aggravated by the activity of RAS,[84,85] independent of, and in addition to, the effect of elevated blood pressure.[86,87] At similar blood pressure levels, incidence of left ventricular hypertrophy was greater with the ARB losartan than with the β-blocker atenolol throughout a follow-up of 5 years.[88–90]

Atrial Fibrillation

Treatment with ARB has been shown to reduce the incidence of atrial fibrillation by 21% in hypertensive patients.[91–93] The mechanism underlying this protective effect is related to the prevention of left atrial dilation and atrial fibrosis and to the reduction of conduction velocity.[81]

Stroke

Several clinical trials have demonstrated a prominent effect of ARB treatment on the prevention of stroke.[88,94–97] At a similar blood pressure, control ARB had an additional 25% reduction in strokes compared with those on a β-blocker.[88] A similar result was also observed in the Study on COgnition and Prognosis in the Elderly (SCOPE).

Atherosclerosis

Activation of RAS through AT1R (1) induces vasoconstriction and formation of extracellular matrix and matrix metalloproteinases, (2) enhances migration and proliferation of vascular smooth muscle cells, (3) increases synthesis of plasminogen activator inhibitor (PAI-1), and (4) stimulates release of proinflammatory cytokines, including IL-6 and TNF-α.[98]

Diabetes

In a meta-analysis, treatment with ARBs has been shown to reduce the incidence of diabetes mellitus by 23%, regardless of the presence of cardiovascular disease.[99–101]

Renal Damage

Treatment with ARBs improves renal damage in patients with and without diabetes.[102–104]

Dementia

Hypertension induces damage to brain microcirculation, which contributes to the development of dementia. However, evidence on the benefit of RAS blockade on cognitive function has been controversial. The role of angiotensin IV on cognitive function has been described.[105–107]

Muscle Strength

A fully functional RAS exists in the skeletal muscle microvasculature. Studies have also confirmed that skeletal muscles generate Ang II locally.[108–110] The polymorphism of the ACE gene is an important factor in determining physical performance.[111] However, clinical studies are needed to confirm a role for blockade of RAS in muscle function.

Osteoporosis, Fracture Risk, and Bone Marrow Density

Clinical studies indicate a possible role of RAS in bone metabolism and fracture risk. Patients treated with an ACE inhibitor showed an increased bone mineral density and a reduced fracture risk.[112–114] In addition, individuals with decreased ACE activity have a higher bone marrow density than individuals with increased ACE activity.[115]

SUMMARY

RAS plays a broad role in vascular regulation, inflammation, oxidative stress, and apoptosis. Each of these molecular realms has been hypothesized to influence the aging phenotype. RAS also clearly influences multiple disease states with increasing age, and pharmaceuticals targeting these pathways are now a mainstay of treatment of many older adults. RAS blockade exerts potent antiatherosclerotic, antihypertensive, antiinflammatory, antiproliferative, and oxidative stress–lowering properties. Given the influence of RAS on frailty-related diseases and traits, and the age-related changes in this system that seem to accelerate these conditions, further evaluation on the causes, multisystemic interactions, and intervention development on RAS regulation is indicated.

REFERENCES

1. Wang M, Takagi G, Asai K, et al. Aging increases aortic MMP-2 activity and angiotensin II in nonhuman primates. Hypertension 2003;41(6):1308–16.
2. Heymes C, Silvestre JS, Llorens-Cortes C, et al. Cardiac senescence is associated with enhanced expression of angiotensin II receptor subtypes. Endocrinology 1998;139(5):2579–87.
3. Min LJ, Mogi M, Iwai M, et al. Signaling mechanisms of angiotensin II in regulating vascular senescence. Ageing Res Rev 2009;8(2):113–21.
4. Chiu AT, McCall DE, Nguyen TT, et al. Discrimination of angiotensin II receptor subtypes by dithiothreitol. Eur J Pharmacol 1989;170(1–2):117–8.
5. Chang RS, Lotti VJ. Two distinct angiotensin II receptor binding sites in rat adrenal revealed by new selective nonpeptide ligands. Mol Pharmacol 1990; 37(3):347–51.
6. Hein L, Barsh GS, Pratt RE, et al. Behavioural and cardiovascular effects of disrupting the angiotensin II type-2 receptor in mice. Nature 1995;377(6551): 744–7.
7. Ichiki T, Labosky PA, Shiota C, et al. Effects on blood pressure and exploratory behaviour of mice lacking angiotensin II type-2 receptor. Nature 1995; 377(6551):748–50.
8. Masaki H, Kurihara T, Yamaki A, et al. Cardiac-specific overexpression of angiotensin II AT2 receptor causes attenuated response to AT1 receptor-mediated pressor and chronotropic effects. J Clin Invest 1998;101(3):527–35.
9. AbdAlla S, Lother H, Abdel-tawab AM, et al. The angiotensin II AT2 receptor is an AT1 receptor antagonist. J Biol Chem 2001;276(43):39721–6.

10. Matsubara H. Pathophysiological role of angiotensin II type 2 receptor in cardiovascular and renal diseases. Circ Res 1998;83(12):1182–91.
11. Bascands JL, Girolami JP, Troly M, et al. Angiotensin II induces phenotype-dependent apoptosis in vascular smooth muscle cells. Hypertension 2001; 38(6):1294–9.
12. Peach MJ. Renin-angiotensin system: biochemistry and mechanisms of action. Physiol Rev 1977;57(2):313–70.
13. Nahmod KA, Vermeulen ME, Raiden S, et al. Control of dendritic cell differentiation by angiotensin II. FASEB J 2003;17(3):491–3.
14. Jurewicz M, McDermott DH, Sechler JM, et al. Human T and natural killer cells possess a functional renin-angiotensin system: further mechanisms of angiotensin II-induced inflammation. J Am Soc Nephrol 2007;18(4):1093–102.
15. Velez JC. The importance of the intrarenal renin-angiotensin system. Nat Clin Pract Nephrol 2009;5(2):89–100.
16. Griendling KK, Ushio-Fukai M, Lassegue B, et al. Angiotensin II signaling in vascular smooth muscle. New concepts. Hypertension 1997;29(1 Pt 2):366–73.
17. Eguchi S, Frank GD, Mifune M, et al. Metalloprotease-dependent ErbB ligand shedding in mediating EGFR transactivation and vascular remodelling. Biochem Soc Trans 2003;31(Pt 6):1198–202.
18. Yin G, Yan C, Berk BC. Angiotensin II signaling pathways mediated by tyrosine kinases. Int J Biochem Cell Biol 2003;35(6):780–3.
19. Suzuki H, Motley ED, Frank GD, et al. Recent progress in signal transduction research of the angiotensin II type-1 receptor: protein kinases, vascular dysfunction and structural requirement. Curr Med Chem Cardiovasc Hematol Agents 2005;3(4):305–22.
20. Steckelings UM, Kaschina E, Unger T. The AT2 receptor–a matter of love and hate. Peptides 2005;26(8):1401–9.
21. Dechend R, Fiebler A, Lindschau C, et al. Modulating angiotensin II-induced inflammation by HMG co-A reductase inhibition. Am J Hypertens 2001; 14(6 Pt 2):55S–61S.
22. Touyz RM, Schiffrin EL. Signal transduction mechanisms mediating the physiological and pathophysiological actions of angiotensin II in vascular smooth muscle cells. Pharmacol Rev 2000;52(4):639–72.
23. Kambayashi Y, Bardhan S, Takahashi K, et al. Molecular cloning of a novel angiotensin II receptor isoform involved in phosphotyrosine phosphatase inhibition. J Biol Chem 1993;268(33):24543–6.
24. Bedecs K, Elbaz N, Sutren M, et al. Angiotensin II type 2 receptors mediate inhibition of mitogen-activated protein kinase cascade and functional activation of SHP-1 tyrosine phosphatase. Biochem J 1997;325(Pt 2):449–54.
25. Horiuchi M, Hayashida W, Kambe T, et al. Angiotensin type 2 receptor dephosphorylates Bcl-2 by activating mitogen-activated protein kinase phosphatase-1 and induces apoptosis. J Biol Chem 1997;272(30):19022–6.
26. Kobori H, Nangaku M, Navar LG, et al. The intrarenal renin-angiotensin system: from physiology to the pathobiology of hypertension and kidney disease. Pharmacol Rev 2007;59(3):251–87.
27. Thompson MM, Oyama TT, Kelly FJ, et al. Activity and responsiveness of the renin-angiotensin system in the aging rat. Am J Physiol Regul Integr Comp Physiol 2000;279(5):R1787–94.
28. Anderson S. Ageing and the renin-angiotensin system. Nephrol Dial Transplant 1997;12(6):1093–4.

29. Anderson S, Rennke HG, Zatz R. Glomerular adaptations with normal aging and with long-term converting enzyme inhibition in rats. Am J Physiol 1994; 267(1 Pt 2):F35–43.
30. Baylis C. Renal responses to acute angiotensin II inhibition and administered angiotensin II in the aging, conscious, chronically catheterized rat. Am J Kidney Dis 1993;22(6):842–50.
31. Baylis C, Corman B. The aging kidney: insights from experimental studies. J Am Soc Nephrol 1998;9(4):699–709.
32. Masilamani S, Zhang XZ, Baylis C. Blunted pressure natriuretic response in the old rat: participation of the renal nerves. Am J Kidney Dis 1998;32(4):605–10.
33. Reckelhoff JF, Baylis C. Proximal tubular metalloprotease activity is decreased in the senescent rat kidney. Life Sci 1992;50(13):959–63.
34. Carey RM, Siragy HM. Newly recognized components of the renin-angiotensin system: potential roles in cardiovascular and renal regulation. Endocr Rev 2003;24(3):261–71.
35. Jones ES, Vinh A, McCarthy CA, et al. AT2 receptors: functional relevance in cardiovascular disease. Pharmacol Ther 2008;120(3):292–316.
36. Widdop RE, Vinh A, Henrion D, et al. Vascular angiotensin AT2 receptors in hypertension and ageing. Clin Exp Pharmacol Physiol 2008;35(4):386–90.
37. Savoia C, Touyz RM, Volpe M, et al. Angiotensin type 2 receptor in resistance arteries of type 2 diabetic hypertensive patients. Hypertension 2007;49(2): 341–6.
38. Warnholtz A, Nickenig G, Schulz E, et al. Increased NADH-oxidase-mediated superoxide production in the early stages of atherosclerosis: evidence for involvement of the renin-angiotensin system. Circulation 1999;99(15):2027–33.
39. Weber MA. Clinical experience with the angiotensin II receptor antagonist losartan. A preliminary report. Am J Hypertens 1992;5(12 Pt 2):247S–51S.
40. Guan H, Cachofeiro V, Pucci ML, et al. Nitric oxide and the depressor response to angiotensin blockade in hypertension. Hypertension 1996;27(1):19–24.
41. Siragy HM, de Gasparo M, Carey RM. Angiotensin type 2 receptor mediates valsartan-induced hypotension in conscious rats. Hypertension 2000;35(5): 1074–7.
42. Oishi Y, Ozono R, Yoshizumi M, et al. AT2 receptor mediates the cardioprotective effects of AT1 receptor antagonist in post-myocardial infarction remodeling. Life Sci 2006;80(1):82–8.
43. Carey RM, Howell NL, Jin XH, et al. Angiotensin type 2 receptor-mediated hypotension in angiotensin type-1 receptor-blocked rats. Hypertension 2001;38(6): 1272–7.
44. Staessen JA, Wang J, Bianchi G, et al. Essential hypertension. Lancet 2003; 361(9369):1629–41.
45. Fraga MF, Ballestar E, Paz MF, et al. Epigenetic differences arise during the lifetime of monozygotic twins. Proc Natl Acad Sci U S A 2005;102(30):10604–9.
46. Gilbert JS, Lang AL, Nijland MJ. Maternal nutrient restriction and the fetal left ventricle: decreased angiotensin receptor expression. Reprod Biol Endocrinol 2005;3:27.
47. Bogdarina I, Welham S, King PJ, et al. Epigenetic modification of the renin-angiotensin system in the fetal programming of hypertension. Circ Res 2007; 100(4):520–6.
48. Ershler WB, Keller ET. Age-associated increased interleukin-6 gene expression, late-life diseases, and frailty. Annu Rev Med 2000;51:245–70.

49. Fujita J, Tsujinaka T, Ebisui C, et al. Role of interleukin-6 in skeletal muscle protein breakdown and cathepsin activity in vivo. Eur Surg Res 1996;28(5): 361–6.
50. Maggio M, Guralnik JM, Longo DL, et al. Interleukin-6 in aging and chronic disease: a magnificent pathway. J Gerontol A Biol Sci Med Sci 2006;61(6): 575–84.
51. Fried LP, Tangen CM, Walston J, et al. Frailty in older adults: evidence for a phenotype. J Gerontol A Biol Sci Med Sci 2001;56(3):M146–56.
52. Walston J, Fried LP. Frailty and the older man. Med Clin North Am 1999;83(5): 1173–94.
53. Chung HY, Cheng KQ, Chung GJ. [Molecular inflammation in aging process]. Nippon Ronen Igakkai Zasshi 2004;41(4):357–64 [in Japanese].
54. Chung HY, Sung B, Jung KJ, et al. The molecular inflammatory process in aging. Antioxid Redox Signal 2006;8(3–4):572–81.
55. Kim HJ, Jung KJ, Yu BP, et al. Modulation of redox-sensitive transcription factors by calorie restriction during aging. Mech Ageing Dev 2002;123(12):1589–95.
56. Ren JL, Pan JS, Lu YP, et al. Inflammatory signaling and cellular senescence. Cell Signal 2009;21(3):378–83.
57. Sasaki M, Ikeda H, Sato Y, et al. Proinflammatory cytokine-induced cellular senescence of biliary epithelial cells is mediated via oxidative stress and activation of ATM pathway: a culture study. Free Radic Res 2008;42(7):625–32.
58. Leng SX, Xue QL, Tian J, et al. Inflammation and frailty in older women. J Am Geriatr Soc 2007;55(6):864–71.
59. Walston J, McBurnie MA, Newman A, et al. Frailty and activation of the inflammation and coagulation systems with and without clinical comorbidities: results from the Cardiovascular Health Study. Arch Intern Med 2002;162(20):2333–41.
60. Cohen HJ, Harris T, Pieper CF. Coagulation and activation of inflammatory pathways in the development of functional decline and mortality in the elderly. Am J Med 2003;114(3):180–7.
61. Suzuki Y, Ruiz-Ortega M, Lorenzo O, et al. Inflammation and angiotensin II. Int J Biochem Cell Biol 2003;35(6):881–900.
62. Nickenig G, Harrison DG. The AT(1)-type angiotensin receptor in oxidative stress and atherogenesis: part I: oxidative stress and atherogenesis. Circulation 2002;105(3):393–6.
63. Cipollone F, Fazia M, Iezzi A, et al. Blockade of the angiotensin II type 1 receptor stabilizes atherosclerotic plaques in humans by inhibiting prostaglandin E2-dependent matrix metalloproteinase activity. Circulation 2004;109(12):1482–8.
64. Navalkar S, Parthasarathy S, Santanam N, et al. Irbesartan, an angiotensin type 1 receptor inhibitor, regulates markers of inflammation in patients with premature atherosclerosis. J Am Coll Cardiol 2001;37(2):440–4.
65. Schieffer B, Schieffer E, Hilfiker-Kleiner D, et al. Expression of angiotensin II and interleukin 6 in human coronary atherosclerotic plaques: potential implications for inflammation and plaque instability. Circulation 2000;101(12):1372–8.
66. Siragy HM, Awad A, Abadir P, et al. The angiotensin II type 1 receptor mediates renal interstitial content of tumor necrosis factor-alpha in diabetic rats. Endocrinology 2003;144(6):2229–33.
67. Tsutamoto T, Wada A, Maeda K, et al. Angiotensin II type 1 receptor antagonist decreases plasma levels of tumor necrosis factor alpha, interleukin-6 and soluble adhesion molecules in patients with chronic heart failure. J Am Coll Cardiol 2000;35(3):714–21.

68. Beasley D. Phorbol ester and interleukin-1 induce interleukin-6 gene expression in vascular smooth muscle cells via independent pathways. J Cardiovasc Pharmacol 1997;29(3):323–30.
69. Han Y, Runge MS, Brasier AR. Angiotensin II induces interleukin-6 transcription in vascular smooth muscle cells through pleiotropic activation of nuclear factor-kappa B transcription factors. Circ Res 1999;84(6):695–703.
70. Hahn AW, Jonas U, Buhler FR, et al. Activation of human peripheral monocytes by angiotensin II. FEBS Lett 1994;347(2–3):178–80.
71. Weidanz JA, Jacobson LM, Muehrer RJ, et al. ATR blockade reduces IFN-gamma production in lymphocytes in vivo and in vitro. Kidney Int 2005;67(6): 2134–42.
72. Abadir PM, Carey RM, Siragy HM. Angiotensin AT2 receptors directly stimulate renal nitric oxide in bradykinin B2-receptor-null mice. Hypertension 2003;42(4): 600–4.
73. Nickenig G, Sachinidis A, Michaelsen F, et al. Upregulation of vascular angiotensin II receptor gene expression by low-density lipoprotein in vascular smooth muscle cells. Circulation 1997;95(2):473–8.
74. Omura T, Yoshiyama M, Takeuchi K, et al. Angiotensin blockade inhibits SIF DNA binding activities via STAT3 after myocardial infarction. J Mol Cell Cardiol 2000;32(1):23–33.
75. Costantino L, Barlocco D. STAT 3 as a target for cancer drug discovery. Curr Med Chem 2008;15(9):834–43.
76. Chappell VL, Le LX, LaGrone L, et al. Stat proteins play a role in tumor necrosis factor alpha gene expression. Shock 2000;14(3):400–2 [discussion: 402–3].
77. Schrader LI, Kinzenbaw DA, Johnson AW, et al. IL-6 deficiency protects against angiotensin II induced endothelial dysfunction and hypertrophy. Arterioscler Thromb Vasc Biol 2007;27(12):2576–81.
78. Wassmann S, Stumpf M, Strehlow K, et al. Interleukin-6 induces oxidative stress and endothelial dysfunction by overexpression of the angiotensin II type 1 receptor. Circ Res 2004;94(4):534–41.
79. Burrell LM, Johnston CI. Angiotensin II receptor antagonists. Potential in elderly patients with cardiovascular disease. Drugs Aging 1997;10(6):421–34.
80. Basso N, Paglia N, Stella I, et al. Protective effect of the inhibition of the renin-angiotensin system on aging. Regul Pept 2005;128(3):247–52.
81. Schmieder RE, Hilgers KF, Schlaich MP, et al. Renin-angiotensin system and cardiovascular risk. Lancet 2007;369(9568):1208–19.
82. Xu J, Carretero OA, Liu YH, et al. Role of AT2 receptors in the cardioprotective effect of AT1 antagonists in mice. Hypertension 2002;40(3):244–50.
83. Jugdutt BI, Menon V. AT2 receptor and apoptosis during AT1 receptor blockade in reperfused myocardial infarction in the rat. Mol Cell Biochem 2004;262(1–2): 203–14.
84. Mancia G, Zanchetti A, Agabiti-Rosei E, et al. Ambulatory blood pressure is superior to clinic blood pressure in predicting treatment-induced regression of left ventricular hypertrophy. SAMPLE Study Group. Study on Ambulatory Monitoring of Blood Pressure and Lisinopril Evaluation. Circulation 1997;95(6):1464–70.
85. Schmieder RE. The role of non-haemodynamic factors of the genesis of LVH. Nephrol Dial Transplant 2005;20(12):2610–2.
86. Mazzolai L, Nussberger J, Aubert JF, et al. Blood pressure-independent cardiac hypertrophy induced by locally activated renin-angiotensin system. Hypertension 1998;31(6):1324–30.

87. Mazzolai L, Pedrazzini T, Nicoud F, et al. Increased cardiac angiotensin II levels induce right and left ventricular hypertrophy in normotensive mice. Hypertension 2000;35(4):985–91.

88. Dahlof B, Devereux RB, Kjeldsen SE, et al. Cardiovascular morbidity and mortality in the losartan intervention for endpoint reduction in hypertension study (LIFE): a randomised trial against atenolol. Lancet 2002;359(9311):995–1003.

89. Lindholm LH, Ibsen H, Dahlof B, et al. Cardiovascular morbidity and mortality in patients with diabetes in the losartan intervention for endpoint reduction in hypertension study (LIFE): a randomised trial against atenolol. Lancet 2002; 359(9311):1004–10.

90. Devereux RB, Dahlof B, Gerdts E, et al. Regression of hypertensive left ventricular hypertrophy by losartan compared with atenolol: the losartan intervention for endpoint reduction in hypertension (LIFE) trial. Circulation 2004;110(11): 1456–62.

91. Wachtell K, Hornestam B, Lehto M, et al. Cardiovascular morbidity and mortality in hypertensive patients with a history of atrial fibrillation: the losartan intervention for end point reduction in hypertension (LIFE) study. J Am Coll Cardiol 2005;45(5):705–11.

92. Wachtell K, Lehto M, Gerdts E, et al. Angiotensin II receptor blockade reduces new-onset atrial fibrillation and subsequent stroke compared to atenolol: the losartan intervention for end point reduction in hypertension (LIFE) study. J Am Coll Cardiol 2005;45(5):712–9.

93. Schmieder RE, Kjeldsen SE, Julius S, et al. Reduced incidence of new-onset atrial fibrillation with angiotensin II receptor blockade: the VALUE trial. J Hypertens 2008;26(3):403–11.

94. Lithell H, Hansson L, Skoog I, et al. The Study on COgnition and Prognosis in the Elderly (SCOPE); outcomes in patients not receiving add-on therapy after randomization. J Hypertens 2004;22(8):1605–12.

95. Lithell H, Hansson L, Skoog I, et al. The Study on COgnition and Prognosis in the Elderly (SCOPE): principal results of a randomized double-blind intervention trial. J Hypertens 2003;21(5):875–86.

96. Skoog I, Lithell H, Hansson L, et al. Effect of baseline cognitive function and antihypertensive treatment on cognitive and cardiovascular outcomes: Study on COgnition and Prognosis in the Elderly (SCOPE). Am J Hypertens 2005;18(8): 1052–9.

97. Chrysant SG. Possible pathophysiologic mechanisms supporting the superior stroke protection of angiotensin receptor blockers compared to angiotensin-converting enzyme inhibitors: clinical and experimental evidence. J Hum Hypertens 2005;19(12):923–31.

98. Farmer JA, Torre-Amione G. The renin angiotensin system as a risk factor for coronary artery disease. Curr Atheroscler Rep 2001;3(2):117–24.

99. Kjeldsen SE, Julius S, Mancia G, et al. Effects of valsartan compared to amlodipine on preventing type 2 diabetes in high-risk hypertensive patients: the VALUE trial. J Hypertens 2006;24(7):1405–12.

100. Scheen AJ. Renin-angiotensin system inhibition prevents type 2 diabetes mellitus. Part 1. A meta-analysis of randomised clinical trials. Diabetes Metab 2004;30(6):487–96.

101. Gillespie EL, White CM, Kardas M, et al. The impact of ACE inhibitors or angiotensin II type 1 receptor blockers on the development of new-onset type 2 diabetes. Diabetes Care 2005;28(9):2261–6.

102. Parving HH, Lehnert H, Brochner-Mortensen J, et al. The effect of irbesartan on the development of diabetic nephropathy in patients with type 2 diabetes. N Engl J Med 2001;345(12):870–8.
103. Lewis EJ, Lewis JB. Treatment of diabetic nephropathy with angiotensin II receptor antagonist. Clin Exp Nephrol 2003;7(1):1–8.
104. Lewis EJ, Hunsicker LG, Clarke WR, et al. Renoprotective effect of the angiotensin-receptor antagonist irbesartan in patients with nephropathy due to type 2 diabetes. N Engl J Med 2001;345(12):851–60.
105. Gard PR. Cognitive-enhancing effects of angiotensin IV. BMC Neurosci 2008; 9(Suppl 2):S15.
106. Wright JW, Harding JW. The brain RAS and Alzheimer's disease. Exp Neurol 2010;223(2):326–33.
107. Wright JW, Harding JW. The angiotensin AT4 receptor subtype as a target for the treatment of memory dysfunction associated with Alzheimer's disease. J Renin Angiotensin Aldosterone Syst 2008;9(4):226–37.
108. Unger T, Gohlke P, Paul M, et al. Tissue renin-angiotensin systems: fact or fiction? J Cardiovasc Pharmacol 1991;18(Suppl 2):S20–5.
109. Atlas SA. The renin-angiotensin system revisited: classical and nonclassical pathway of angiotensin formation. Mt Sinai J Med 1998;65(2):87–96.
110. Danser AH. Local renin-angiotensin systems. Mol Cell Biochem 1996;157(1–2): 211–6.
111. Montgomery H, Clarkson P, Barnard M, et al. Angiotensin-converting-enzyme gene insertion/deletion polymorphism and response to physical training. Lancet 1999;353(9152):541–5.
112. Perez-Castrillon JL, Justo I, Silva J, et al. Relationship between bone mineral density and angiotensin converting enzyme polymorphism in hypertensive postmenopausal women. Am J Hypertens 2003;16(3):233–5.
113. Perez-Castrillon JL, Silva J, Justo I, et al. Effect of quinapril, quinapril-hydrochlorothiazide, and enalapril on the bone mass of hypertensive subjects: relationship with angiotensin converting enzyme polymorphisms. Am J Hypertens 2003;16(6):453–9.
114. Rejnmark L, Vestergaard P, Mosekilde L. Treatment with beta-blockers, ACE inhibitors, and calcium-channel blockers is associated with a reduced fracture risk: a nationwide case-control study. J Hypertens 2006;24(3):581–9.
115. Woods D, Onambele G, Woledge R, et al. Angiotensin-I converting enzyme genotype-dependent benefit from hormone replacement therapy in isometric muscle strength and bone mineral density. J Clin Endocrinol Metab 2001; 86(5):2200–4.

Anemia in Frailty

Cindy N. Roy, PhD

KEYWORDS

- Anemia • Frailty • Hemoglobin • Disability
- Older adult • Inflammation

PREVALENCE OF ANEMIA IN OLDER ADULTS

The purpose of this article is to highlight the problem of anemia in a challenging population of patients, often referred to as the frail elderly. This population of older adults often live in the community, as opposed to residential facilities for older adults. Hence, the focus of this article is on data gathered in community-dwelling older adults **(Table 1)**. With the establishment of criteria from the World Health Organization (WHO),[1] anemia is usually defined as hemoglobin less than 13 g/dL for men and less than 12 g/dL for women. These criteria are based on values collected from average individuals with no underlying disease. Using these criteria, a study of the third National Health and Nutrition Examination survey (NHANES 1991–1994) found that 10.2% of community-dwelling adults more than 65 years of age were anemic.[2] The incidence of anemia more than doubles to more than 20% in adults more than 85 years of age in the same survey. This is consistent with the general prevalence of anemia reported earlier in the Leiden 85-plus Study,[3] the Cardiovascular Health Study,[4] and the Established Populations for Epidemiologic Studies of the Elderly (EPESE).[5,6] These studies further showed that a greater percentage of men develop anemia late in life than women[2,3] and that anemia affects non-Hispanic blacks at a rate nearly 3 times greater than in non-Hispanic whites.[2,4–6]

In addition to using the WHO-defined criteria for anemia, another approach to establish the ideal hemoglobin value in a population is to assay a selected population for the variable in question. This approach was used by Milman and colleagues[7] who determined hemoglobin concentration in 358 80-year-old Danes. In practice, this selects for a population of older adults that has successfully survived 80 years. They determined the average hemoglobin for 80-year-old men to be 14.0 g/dL and for 80-year-old women to be 13.1 g/dL, higher than the values defined by the WHO. Using the WHO anemia criteria, the prevalence of anemia in this Danish population of adults 80 years of age was similar (17%–18%) to that found for NHANES III adults

---

This work was supported by the American Society for Hematology Scholar Program, the Nathan and Margaret Shock Foundation, the Johns Hopkins University Older American's Independence Center (P30 AG021334), and R01 DK082722.

Division of Geriatric Medicine and Gerontology, Department of Medicine, Johns Hopkins University School of Medicine, 5501 Hopkins Bayview Circle, Baltimore, MD 21224, USA

E-mail address: Croy6@jhmi.edu

Clin Geriatr Med 27 (2011) 67–78
doi:10.1016/j.cger.2010.08.005
0749-0690/11/$ – see front matter © 2011 Elsevier Inc. All rights reserved.

Table 1
Population-based study groups important to anemia of aging

Study	Abbreviation	Location	Participants	Ages	References
Baltimore Longitudinal Study on Aging	BLSA	Baltimore, MD	1400	20 years +	71
Cardiovascular Health Study	CHS	United States	5888	65 years +	4
Chicago Health Aging Project	CHAP	Chicago, IL	1806	65 years +	12
Established Populations for Epidemiologic Studies of the Elderly	EPESE	United States	3607	71 years +	5,6
Invecchiare in Chianti	InCHIANTI	Chianti, Italy	1156	65 years +	9,17,20,70,80
Leiden 85-plus Study	Leiden	Leiden, the Netherlands	1258	85 years +	3
Milman Study	N/A	Denmark	359	80 years	7
Third National Health and Nutrition Examination Survey	NHANES III	United States	4199	65 years +	2
Women's Health and Aging Study	WHAS	Baltimore, MD	1002	65 years +	8,10,11,18

more than 85 years of age. The investigators concluded that optimal hemoglobin concentrations for older adults may be higher than the WHO cut-off for anemia. This has led to concern that the WHO hemoglobin cut-off is not sufficient when screening vulnerable older adults, as discussed in the next section.

CONSEQUENCES OF ANEMIA IN OLDER ADULTS AND IN FRAILTY

Low hemoglobin levels, independent of other health conditions, put older adults at risk for several adverse health outcomes associated with poor oxygen delivery including exhaustion, fatigue,[8] failing muscle strength,[9] and cognitive decline.[5,10] The increased mortality risk for older adults with anemia is well documented.[3–6,11,12] This risk is not accounted for by underlying disease,[3,4,6] suggesting anemia, alone, is a risk factor for death in older adults. Several of these studies also provide evidence that older adults who are not anemic by WHO standards, but have low to normal hemoglobin levels, still have higher mortality risk than nonanemic controls.[4,6,11] Frailty has been associated with being African-American,[13] and because anemia is more likely to affect non-Hispanic black older adults,[2,6] several investigators have looked more closely at anemia as a predictor of mortality for either blacks or whites. A recent follow-up study assessed the relationship between hemoglobin concentration and a significant increase in the risk of death in both race groups in NHANES III.[14] The investigators concluded that the risk of death for non-Hispanic blacks increases significantly at 0.7 g/dL less than the WHO-defined hemoglobin limit, whereas the risk of death for non-Hispanic whites is 0.4 g/dL higher than the WHO-defined limit. The difference in hemoglobin concentration for the mortality signal in these 2 groups is similar to the overall difference in average hemoglobin between these groups, and was not explained by variability in the cause or type of anemia. Similar results were reported for mortality of anemic black and white older adults in Chicago.[12] These findings support more specific stratified criteria for anemia in older adults based on race, in addition to gender, and are especially important to consider when designing studies to treat anemia in these groups.

To investigate the effect of anemia on adverse clinical outcomes before death, Chaves and colleagues[8] assessed whether the WHO anemia criteria also identified women at risk for mobility difficulty. Using self-reported mobility difficulty scores and a performance-based summary score obtained from the Women's Health and Aging Study, the investigators showed that mobility scores improved for women as hemoglobin concentrations increased from 12 to 14 g/dL. They concluded that a hemoglobin level of 12 or even 13 g/dL might not be sufficient for identifying women at risk for disability. Similarly, the prevalence of frailty in the Cardiovascular Health Study significantly increased as hemoglobin levels declined, even though hemoglobin concentration remained higher than the WHO cut-off for anemia.[4]

Strong relationships exist between anemia and the expected physiologic effects of reduced hemoglobin concentration, such as reduced physical performance, fatigue, and declining muscle strength in the elderly.[15] Low to normal hemoglobin level higher than the WHO cut-off was associated with decreased hand-grip strength, fatigue, and decreased quality of life in older community-dwelling adults in the United States.[16] Anemic older adults were found to have lower muscle strength[9,17] and lower muscle density[17] than nonanemic controls in the InCHIANTI study. Even measurable declines in executive function[10] and cognitive impairment[18] are associated with anemia in older women.

Given that anemia affects between 10% and 20% of older adults and given that anemia is closely associated with impaired cognition, fatigue, disability, and mortality, the identification of effective strategies for the treatment of anemia in older adults seems to be an area worthy of intense biomedical investigation. However, most of the data is epidemiologic in nature and does not prove a causal role for anemia with respect to these poor health outcomes. Randomized, controlled clinical trials to improve hemoglobin concentration might provide evidence for a causal role and may positively affect physical performance and quality of life for older adults. Unfortunately, such studies have been severely hindered because the underlying cause of anemia in older adults varies widely and, most often, cannot be easily treated.

PATHOGENESIS OF ANEMIA IN OLDER ADULTS

Approximately one-third of the anemia diagnosed in the NHANES study[2] could be attributed to nutrient deficiencies (iron, vitamin B_{12}, and folate), another third attributed to chronic inflammation (renal disease 12%, chronic inflammation 24%), and the final third had no explained cause. The results were consistent with an earlier study of adults admitted to an acute geriatric ward that identified anemia of chronic inflammation in 35% of patients,[19] and with findings from the InCHIANTI study.[20] Because diagnostic and treatment algorithms for nutrient deficiencies are commonly used in clinical practice settings (**Table 2**), most of this article focuses on the pathogenesis of anemias that are more likely to affect frail, older adults, namely anemia related to inflammation and anemia of unclear cause.

Frail older adults have poorer health status than robust older adults, more chronic diseases, and more comorbid conditions.[13] Active low-grade inflammation is, therefore, a common finding in the frail elderly.[21] Activation of nuclear factor kappa B (NFkB) is the hallmark of chronic inflammation, making NFkB and its transcriptional target genes (**Fig. 1**) prime candidates for interventions against frailty and pathophysiologic outcomes related to frailty, such as anemia. NFkB drives transcription of multiple inflammatory biomediators such as interleukin-6 (IL-6) and chemokines that

Table 2
Clinical diagnostic tests important in the diagnosis of anemia in older adults

Test	Pathogenic	Discriminates	References
Mean cell volume (MCV)	>100 fL <80 fL	Iron vs B_{12}/folate deficiency Iron deficiency vs AICD	31
Mean cell hemoglobin (MCH)	<27 pg or >31 pg	Iron deficiency vs AICD	
Vitamin B_{12}	<200 pg/mL	Macrocytic anemia	2
Folate	RBC: <102.6 ng/mL Serum: <2.6 ng/mL	Macrocytic anemia	2
Serum iron	<60 µg/dL	Iron deficiency/AICD vs unexplained anemia	59
Transferrin saturation (TS)	<15%	Iron deficiency/AICD vs unexplained anemia	68,81
Serum ferritin (sFt)	<12 ng/mL	Iron deficiency vs AICD	2,82
Soluble transferrin receptor/log(serum ferritin) (sTfR/log sFt)	>1.5 >0.8	Iron deficiency vs AICD AICD with iron deficiency anemia	81
Estimated creatinine clearance (eCC)	<30 mL/min	AICD vs anemia of chronic kidney disease	83
C-reactive protein (CRP)	>10 mg/dL	Iron deficiency vs AICD	

Abbreviations: AICD, anemia of inflammation or chronic disease; RBC, red blood cells.

promote the clearance of infection and the healing of wounds.[22,23] Increasingly, genes and proteins recognized for their ability to promote longevity have been shown to dampen NFkB activity, indicating a molecular link between aging biology and chronic inflammation.

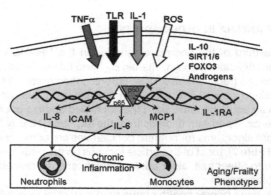

Fig. 1. Overview of NFkB and chronic inflammation. Type I acute phase cytokines, tumor necrosis factor α (TNFα), interleukin-1 (IL-1); signaling through the toll-like receptors (TLR); and reactive oxygen species (ROS) all induce translocation of NFkB (p65/p50) to the nucleus where it induces transcription of the chemokines IL-8 and monocyte chemoattractant protein 1 (MCP1) as well as the proinflammatory cytokine IL-6. Increased circulating neutrophils, increased circulating monocytes, and increased IL-6 are all markers of aging and a central piece of the frailty phenotype. (*Courtesy of* Cindy N. Roy, PhD, Baltimore, MD.)

The mammalian longevity gene, SIRT1, deacetylates NFkB and prevents transcription of its target genes.[24] SIRT6 has also been shown to inhibit NFkB-mediated gene expression.[25] FOXO3A is implicated in the regulation of NFkB inhibitors,[26] and estrogen[27] and testosterone[28] have also been shown to inhibit NFkB activity. Global expression of NFkB gene targets were recently shown to increase with chronologic age in both humans and mice.[29] Increased free radicals, which accumulate with age, also activate NFkB and inflammation.[30] These data suggest that chronic inflammation driven by NFkB may promote specific poor health outcomes in frail older adults. In the next sections, the potential mechanisms by which inflammation might promote anemia in the frail elderly are investigated.

IL-6 and Anemia

Given their chronic proinflammatory state, much of the anemia in the frail elderly is consistent with anemia of inflammation or chronic disease (AICD). AICD is most often described as a normocytic, normochromic anemia, but in severe cases, AICD can become microcytic and hypochromic.[31] AICD is characterized by some combination of iron restriction, insufficient marrow response to the anemia, and decreased erythrocyte survival.[31] Significantly increased serum C-reactive protein (CRP) and IL-6 levels in frail patients clearly indicate a low-grade, chronic proinflammatory phenotype. The serum concentrations of these inflammatory markers are many orders of magnitude lower than concentrations achieved during acute infection, yet the physiology of frail older adults suggests that even low concentrations affect key biologic systems,[32] including the erythron. Understanding how specific cytokines regulate erythrocyte production and turnover will uncover new pathways that may serve as targets for novel anemia treatment strategies in the frail elderly. Progress in this field has been limited by a poor understanding of the key inflammatory mediators that drive anemia in general.

Recently, compelling evidence has emerged supporting the relationship between anemia and IL-6, which has been dubbed "the cytokine for gerontologists."[33] IL-6 correlates best with anemia in several disease states. In the elderly, frail older adults in particular, anemia is most closely associated with increased IL-6.[34–36] Nikolaisen and colleagues[37] measured IL-1β, IL-2, IL-6, IL-8, and TNFα in patients with rheumatoid arthritis with and without anemia and found that IL-6 levels were highest in the anemic group. IL-6 was the only cytokine of those tested that negatively correlated with hemoglobin concentration. IL-6 was also found to be more significantly increased in anemic patients than in nonanemic patients with systemic lupus erythematosus.[38] The same study found a negative correlation between hemoglobin and IL-6. Although no causality can be proved from these population studies, they provide important evidence that the mechanisms underlying AICD and anemia associated with frailty may be conserved.

IL-6 has been shown to specifically downregulate beta globin mRNA in burst-forming unit-E cultures,[39] which would be expected to decrease hemoglobin production. The observation that erythrocyte numbers increase and platelet numbers decrease after prolonged hypoxia, has led many investigators to hypothesize that stem cell competition, or limited proliferative capacity of megakaryocyte-erythrocyte progenitors, may explain these phenomena.[40–42] Because erythrocyte numbers decrease and platelet numbers increase in the context of inflammation, inflammatory cytokines may similarly encourage cell fate. IL-6 induces thrombocytosis in primates and simultaneously reduces the number of red blood cells.[43–45] However, IL-6 seems to stimulate increased platelet production from conserved numbers of megakaryocytes.[46] IL-6 may, therefore, have independent effects on later-stage erythroid and platelet precursors. Interactions between IL-6, erythrocytes, and platelet numbers become important in considering interventions for improving anemia and the factors that might promote adverse events, such as thromboembolism, in response to interventional therapy.

In addition to the potential for direct effects of IL-6 on erythroid precursors, IL-6 orchestrates the type II acute phase response that restricts iron availability by inducing the expression of factors including serum ceruloplasmin (Cp)[47] and hepcidin antimicrobial peptide (Hepc).[48] As both Cp and Hepc regulate iron delivery to the erythron, they strongly affect hemoglobin production and the final stages of erythroid development.

Peripheral White Cells and Anemia in Frail Older Adults

NFkB also promotes transcription of chemokines such as IL-8 and monocyte chemoattractant protein 1 (MCP1), which facilitate homing of neutrophils and monocytes to sites of tissue injury or infection. Recently, increased circulating neutrophil and monocytes counts have been associated with frailty, independent of IL-6.[49] Whether the appearance of such inflammatory cells in frail older adults indicates peripheral tissue injury resulting from underlying disease or the consequence of dysregulated chemokine expression, courtesy of NFkB, remains to be seen. In either case, oxidative stress levels can be expected to be higher in individuals with higher numbers of circulating inflammatory cells. Anemia has been linked to increased oxidative stress in several experimental and disease states.[50-53] Because the primary role of an erythrocyte is to carry oxygen, many enzymes that scavenge reactive oxygen species are expressed in terminally differentiated erythrocytes.[52] When these enzymes are overwhelmed in their capacity to scavenge reactive oxygen species, erythrocyte life span is reduced and eventually anemia can result.[51,52]

A striking example of the important relationship between antioxidant capacity and anemia has come from WHAS I and II and NHANES III. In both cohorts,[54,55] anemia was strongly associated with low levels of serum selenium. Individuals with anemia from nutritional causes, inflammation, or unexplained causes were more likely to have low selenium levels. Selenium is a critical cofactor for antioxidant enzymes such as glutathione peroxidase,[56] which is highly expressed in erythrocytes.[52] Thus, selenium deficiency in older adults is likely to exacerbate anemia related to multiple causes.

ANEMIA OF UNEXPLAINED CAUSE

The NHANES III study, which investigated anemia in older adults, determined that one-third of anemia in older adults could not be explained using the diagnostic tests and criteria available.[2] Any individual with anemia and normal nutrients (serum iron, folate and vitamin B_{12}) would be in this category. Studies in other community-based populations have also identified a significant proportion of patients whose anemia cannot be clearly diagnosed with available diagnostic criteria.[57,58] Generally speaking, such unexplained anemia tends to be mild and normocytic with normal iron parameters.[59] Although the anemia is unexplained or unclear, many known biologic processes that occur with age may contribute, individually or in combination, to this anemia.[59,60] Such biologic processes might include erythropoietin insufficiency[20,61]; androgen insufficiency[27,28]; alterations in erythroid progenitors, hematopoietic stem cells, and their bone marrow niche[62-64]; hypoxia sensing[65,66]; inflammation,[36] or development of myelodysplastic syndrome.[67]

The knowledge regarding these possible causes in large numbers of healthy or frail humans is scant because they require advanced technology for analysis or because they are difficult to assess in the bone marrow of frail elderly. Sufficient levels of erythropoietin (Epo) are critical for maintenance of red blood cell numbers. Epo is primarily produced by the kidney, so in the context of mild renal disease, low Epo levels may be suspected.[58] Many older adults with unexplained anemia and no evidence of inflammation have low Epo levels,[20] thus routine analysis of serum Epo concentration in anemic older adults may be useful. In addition, inflammation can suppress erythropoietic drive.[68] Inflammatory markers such as CRP, specific proinflammatory cytokines, and Hepc should be investigated. Myelodysplastic syndrome, a bone marrow failure syndrome, is common in older adults. Often, pancytopenia, including anemia, is an initial feature that may transform to leukemia.[69] Bone marrow biopsy to assess dysplastic changes in multiple hematopoetic cell lines is essential for a definitive diagnosis of myelodysplastic syndrome. Because frail older adults often have multiple chronic diseases and a poor aging phenotype, it would not be surprising to find mutifactorial causes for their anemia. Continued collaboration between large epidemiologic studies and molecular hematologists will remain a requirement for successful analyses and for advancing our knowledge of anemia in the frail elderly.

INTERVENTIONS FOR CONSIDERATION

An extensive evidence base concerning the problem of anemia in the elderly has developed in the last decade. However, most of the evidence is epidemiologic in nature and does not support causal relationships between anemia and poor health outcomes. This section addresses the areas of research that would extend our clinical and basic biology evidence base toward appropriate diagnostic tools and feasible interventions or preventative measures against anemia in frail older adults. The diagnostics or pharmacologic agents outlined lack sufficient evidence to be appropriately indicated for treatment of anemia in the frail elderly or accepted as part of standard clinical practice. Anemia is most often treated in the elderly when the hemoglobin level falls sufficiently low to require transfusion.

Frail older adults share a proinflammatory phenotype without regard to underlying disease status. Much of the anemia observed in this population is likely to be the result of chronic inflammation, but standard clinical practice does not use the most sensitive assays (eg, IL-6 ELISA) that would diagnose chronic inflammation. In principle, anemia associated with chronic inflammation is treated when the underlying disease is successfully treated. However, for frail older adults, the underlying disease often cannot be resolved. Because anemia is strongly associated with impaired cognition, fatigue, disability, and mortality in older adults, independent of disease state, the medical community must consider the safety and efficacy of anemia treatment of the frail elderly in the absence of a direct diagnosis of disease. As such, the rigor with which anemia is assessed in the elderly must be increased and new strategies must be tested for their ability to successfully predict patients who will benefit from treatment.

For older adults without the diagnosis of a chronic inflammatory disease or infection and no evidence of nutrient deficiencies, erythropoietin-stimulating agents (ESAs) may seem like a plausible option for treatment of anemia. Many anemic older adults have lower Epo concentrations that nonanemic controls.[70] However, Epo levels tend to increase with age even when hemoglobin levels decrease,[71] suggesting the problem is not production of Epo, but an effective response to it. The serious nature of off-target effects of recombinant human Epo,[72–74] including myocardial infarction and stroke, usually preclude the use of this potential intervention in the frail elderly. One randomized, placebo-controlled, clinical trial has shown that ESAs can be used safely and effectively in older adults.[61] However, without specific guidelines for their use in the frail elderly and without strong evidence for improved quality of life with treatment, ESAs remain an unpalatable choice for most geriatric patients.

Inhibition of hemoglobin production by IL-6 is likely to be a key step in the pathophysiology of anemia in frail older adults that could be targeted by novel treatments. Hemoglobin synthesis occurs after Epo is required. Treatment options that target hemoglobin production independent of Epo are especially relevant considering the serious adverse events associated with ESA use. Modulators of the IL-6 signaling pathway, such as tocilizumab, are available. However, this class of drugs has mild to moderate complications including infusion reactions, liver dysfunction, and infections.[75] Another drawback to interventions that specifically target IL-6 is that IL-6 is only one part of a widespread inflammatory response in most frail patients. Identification of an intervention that targets inflammation more broadly may be more beneficial to this population.

Agents that target NFkB would certainly provide broad spectrum inhibition of inflammatory mediators. Aspirin and salicylates prevent activation of NFkB,[76] making them potentially very useful. However, the use of aspirin and nonsteroidal antiinflammatory drugs is associated with gastrointestinal bleeding.[77] Nonacetylated salicylates, such as salsalate, inhibit NFkB activity and have a smaller risk of bleeding.[78,79] Epidemiologic studies investigating the relationship between the use of nonacetylated salicylates and outcomes such as anemia and frailty and randomized controlled trials would be useful to assess the feasibility of this drug class to improve anemia and quality of life for frail older adults.

SUMMARY

The last decade has produced an overwhelming amount of epidemiologic evidence that indicates anemic older adults are at risk for impaired cognition, fatigue, disability, and death. However, sufficient evidence from randomized controlled trials that supports a causative role for anemia associated with functional decline and death does not exist. Justified subject and Institutional Review Board resistance to clinical trials and poorly defined pathogenesis of anemia in the elderly pose significant barriers to the development of informative randomized controlled trials. Studies in the frail elderly should focus on the role of the inflammatory process in the pathogenesis of anemia. Outcomes and end points in clinical trials should focus on specific indicators of physical function such as grip strength, walking speed, or timed up-and-go rather than on hemoglobin concentration alone. Investing material resources and expertise in the development of new strategies and practices for the diagnosis, treatment, and prevention of anemia in the elderly will surely result in improved quality of care and improved quality of life for 1 of the most vulnerable groups in society.

REFERENCES

1. Nutritional anaemias. Report of a WHO scientific group. World Health Organ Tech Rep Ser 1968;405:5–37.
2. Guralnik JM, Eisenstaedt RS, Ferrucci L, et al. Prevalence of anemia in persons 65 years and older in the United States: evidence for a high rate of unexplained anemia. Blood 2004;104(8):2263–8.
3. Izaks GJ, Westendorp RG, Knook DL. The definition of anemia in older persons. JAMA 1999;281(18):1714–7.

4. Zakai NA, Katz R, Hirsch C, et al. A prospective study of anemia status, hemoglobin concentration, and mortality in an elderly cohort: the Cardiovascular Health Study. Arch Intern Med 2005;165(19):2214–20.

5. Denny SD, Kuchibhatla MN, Cohen HJ. Impact of anemia on mortality, cognition, and function in community-dwelling elderly. Am J Med 2006;119(4):327–34.

6. Penninx BW, Pahor M, Woodman RC, et al. Anemia in old age is associated with increased mortality and hospitalization. J Gerontol A Biol Sci Med Sci 2006;61(5): 474–9.

7. Milman N, Pedersen AN, Ovesen L, et al. Hemoglobin concentrations in 358 apparently healthy 80-year-old Danish men and women. Should the reference interval be adjusted for age? Aging Clin Exp Res 2008;20(1):8–14.

8. Chaves PH, Ashar B, Guralnik JM, et al. Looking at the relationship between hemoglobin concentration and prevalent mobility difficulty in older women. Should the criteria currently used to define anemia in older people be reevaluated? J Am Geriatr Soc 2002;50(7):1257–64.

9. Penninx BW, Pahor M, Cesari M, et al. Anemia is associated with disability and decreased physical performance and muscle strength in the elderly. J Am Geriatr Soc 2004;52(5):719–24.

10. Chaves PH, Carlson MC, Ferrucci L, et al. Association between mild anemia and executive function impairment in community-dwelling older women: the Women's Health and Aging Study II. J Am Geriatr Soc 2006;54(9):1429–35.

11. Chaves PH, Xue QL, Guralnik JM, et al. What constitutes normal hemoglobin concentration in community-dwelling disabled older women? J Am Geriatr Soc 2004;52(11):1811–6.

12. Dong X, Mendes de Leon C, Artz A, et al. A population-based study of hemoglobin, race, and mortality in elderly persons. J Gerontol A Biol Sci Med Sci 2008;63(8):873–8.

13. Fried LP, Tangen CM, Walston J, et al. Frailty in older adults: evidence for a phenotype. J Gerontol A Biol Sci Med Sci 2001;56(3):M146–56.

14. Patel KV, Longo DL, Ershler WB, et al. Haemoglobin concentration and the risk of death in older adults: differences by race/ethnicity in the NHANES III follow-up. Br J Haematol 2009;145(4):514–23.

15. Artz AS. Anemia and the frail elderly. Semin Hematol 2008;45(4):261–6.

16. Thein M, Ershler WB, Artz AS, et al. Diminished quality of life and physical function in community-dwelling elderly with anemia. Medicine 2009;88(2):107–14.

17. Cesari M, Penninx BW, Lauretani F, et al. Hemoglobin levels and skeletal muscle: results from the InCHIANTI study. J Gerontol A Biol Sci Med Sci 2004;59(3): 249–54.

18. Deal JA, Carlson MC, Xue QL, et al. Anemia and 9-year domain-specific cognitive decline in community-dwelling older women: the Women's Health and Aging Study II. J Am Geriatr Soc 2009;57(9):1604–11.

19. Joosten E, Pelemans W, Hiele M, et al. Prevalence and causes of anaemia in a geriatric hospitalized population. Gerontology 1992;38(1–2):111–7.

20. Ferrucci L, Guralnik JM, Bandinelli S, et al. Unexplained anaemia in older persons is characterised by low erythropoietin and low levels of pro-inflammatory markers. Br J Haematol 2007;136(6):849–55.

21. Walston J, McBurnie MA, Newman A, et al. Frailty and activation of the inflammation and coagulation systems with and without clinical comorbidities: results from the Cardiovascular Health Study. Arch Intern Med 2002;162(20):2333–41.

22. Hanada T, Yoshimura A. Regulation of cytokine signaling and inflammation. Cytokine Growth Factor Rev 2002;13(4–5):413–21.

23. Ghosh S, Hayden MS. New regulators of NF-kappaB in inflammation. Nat Rev Immunol 2008;8(11):837–48.
24. Yeung F, Hoberg JE, Ramsey CS, et al. Modulation of NF-kappaB-dependent transcription and cell survival by the SIRT1 deacetylase. EMBO J 2004;23(12):2369–80.
25. Kawahara TL, Michishita E, Adler AS, et al. SIRT6 links histone H3 lysine 9 deacetylation to NF-kappaB-dependent gene expression and organismal life span. Cell 2009;136(1):62–74.
26. Lin L, Hron JD, Peng SL. Regulation of NF-kappaB, Th activation, and autoinflammation by the forkhead transcription factor Foxo3a. Immunity 2004;21(2):203–13.
27. Sun WH, Keller ET, Stebler BS, et al. Estrogen inhibits phorbol ester-induced I kappa B alpha transcription and protein degradation. Biochem Biophys Res Commun 1998;244(3):691–5.
28. Keller ET, Chang C, Ershler WB. Inhibition of NFkappaB activity through maintenance of IkappaBalpha levels contributes to dihydrotestosterone-mediated repression of the interleukin-6 promoter. J Biol Chem 1996;271(42):26267–75.
29. Adler AS, Kawahara TL, Segal E, et al. Reversal of aging by NFkappaB blockade. Cell Cycle 2008;7(5):556–9.
30. Yu BP, Chung HY. Adaptive mechanisms to oxidative stress during aging. Mech Ageing Dev 2006;127(5):436–43.
31. Cartwright GE. The anemia of chronic disorders. Semin Hematol 1966;3:351–75.
32. Leng SX, Xue QL, Tian J, et al. Inflammation and frailty in older women. J Am Geriatr Soc 2007;55(6):864–71.
33. Ershler WB. Interleukin-6: a cytokine for gerontologists. J Am Geriatr Soc 1993; 41(2):176–81.
34. Eisenstaedt R, Penninx BW, Woodman RC. Anemia in the elderly: current understanding and emerging concepts. Blood Rev 2006;20(4):213–26.
35. Ershler WB. Biological interactions of aging and anemia: a focus on cytokines. J Am Geriatr Soc 2003;51(Suppl 3):S18–21.
36. Leng S, Chaves P, Koenig K, et al. Serum interleukin-6 and hemoglobin as physiological correlates in the geriatric syndrome of frailty: a pilot study. J Am Geriatr Soc 2002;50(7):1268–71.
37. Nikolaisen C, Figenschau Y, Nossent JC. Anemia in early rheumatoid arthritis is associated with interleukin 6-mediated bone marrow suppression, but has no effect on disease course or mortality. J Rheumatol 2008;35(3):380–6.
38. Ripley BJ, Goncalves B, Isenberg DA, et al. Raised levels of interleukin 6 in systemic lupus erythematosus correlate with anaemia. Ann Rheum Dis 2005; 64(6):849–53.
39. Ferry AE, Baliga SB, Monteiro C, et al. Globin gene silencing in primary erythroid cultures. An inhibitory role for interleukin-6. J Biol Chem 1997;272(32):20030–7.
40. McDonald TP, Clift RE, Cottrell MB. Large, chronic doses of erythropoietin cause thrombocytopenia in mice. Blood 1992;80(2):352–8.
41. Beguin Y. Erythropoietin and platelet production. Haematologica 1999;84(6):541–7.
42. Lu J, Guo S, Ebert BL, et al. MicroRNA-mediated control of cell fate in megakaryocyte-erythrocyte progenitors. Dev Cell 2008;14(6):843–53.
43. Hill RJ, Warren MK, Levin J. Stimulation of thrombopoiesis in mice by human recombinant interleukin 6. J Clin Invest 1990;85(4):1242–7.
44. Asano S, Okano A, Ozawa K, et al. In vivo effects of recombinant human interleukin-6 in primates: stimulated production of platelets. Blood 1990;75(8):1602–5.
45. Sun WH, Binkley N, Bidwell DW, et al. The influence of recombinant human interleukin-6 on blood and immune parameters in middle-aged and old rhesus monkeys. Lymphokine Cytokine Res 1993;12(6):449–55.

46. An E, Ogata K, Kuriya S, et al. Interleukin-6 and erythropoietin act as direct poten-
    tiators and inducers of in vitro cytoplasmic process formation on purified mouse
    megakaryocytes. Exp Hematol 1994;22(2):149–56.
47. Ramadori G, Van Damme J, Rieder H, et al. Interleukin 6, the third mediator of
    acute-phase reaction, modulates hepatic protein synthesis in human and mouse.
    Comparison with interleukin 1 beta and tumor necrosis factor-alpha. Eur J Immu-
    nol 1988;18(8):1259–64.
48. Nemeth E, Valore EV, Territo M, et al. Hepcidin, a putative mediator of anemia of
    inflammation, is a type II acute-phase protein. Blood 2003;101(7):2461–3.
49. Leng SX, Xue QL, Tian J, et al. Associations of neutrophil and monocyte counts
    with frailty in community-dwelling disabled older women: results from the
    Women's Health and Aging Studies I. Exp Gerontol 2009;44(8):511–6.
50. Friedman JS, Lopez MF, Fleming MD, et al. SOD2-deficiency anemia: protein
    oxidation and altered protein expression reveal targets of damage, stress
    response, and antioxidant responsiveness. Blood 2004;104(8):2565–73.
51. Lyons BL, Lynes MA, Burzenski L, et al. Mechanisms of anemia in SHP-1 protein
    tyrosine phosphatase-deficient "viable motheaten" mice. Exp Hematol 2003;
    31(3):234–43.
52. Marinkovic D, Zhang X, Yalcin S, et al. Foxo3 is required for the regulation of
    oxidative stress in erythropoiesis. J Clin Invest 2007;117(8):2133–44.
53. Rocha-Pereira P, Santos-Silva A, Rebelo I, et al. Erythrocyte damage in mild and
    severe psoriasis. Br J Dermatol 2004;150(2):232–44.
54. Semba RD, Ferrucci L, Cappola AR, et al. Low serum selenium is associated with
    anemia among older women living in the community: the Women's Health and
    Aging Studies I and II. Biol Trace Elem Res 2006;112(2):97–107.
55. Semba RD, Ricks MO, Ferrucci L, et al. Low serum selenium is associated with
    anemia among older adults in the United States. Eur J Clin Nutr 2009;63(1):93–9.
56. Lu J, Holmgren A. Selenoproteins. J Biol Chem 2009;284(2):723–7.
57. Ania BJ, Suman VJ, Fairbanks VF, et al. Incidence of anemia in older people: an
    epidemiologic study in a well defined population. J Am Geriatr Soc 1997;45(7):
    825–31.
58. Ble A, Fink JC, Woodman RC, et al. Renal function, erythropoietin, and anemia of
    older persons: the InCHIANTI study. Arch Intern Med 2005;165(19):2222–7.
59. Makipour S, Kanapuru B, Ershler WB. Unexplained anemia in the elderly. Semin
    Hematol 2008;45(4):250–4.
60. Price EA. Aging and erythropoiesis: current state of knowledge. Blood Cells Mol
    Dis 2008;41(2):158–65.
61. Agnihotri P, Telfer M, Butt Z, et al. Chronic anemia and fatigue in elderly patients:
    results of a randomized, double-blind, placebo-controlled, crossover exploratory
    study with epoetin alfa. J Am Geriatr Soc 2007;55(10):1557–65.
62. Gazit R, Weissman IL, Rossi DJ. Hematopoietic stem cells and the aging hema-
    topoietic system. Semin Hematol 2008;45(4):218–24.
63. Chambers SM, Goodell MA. Hematopoietic stem cell aging: wrinkles in stem cell
    potential. Stem Cell Rev 2007;3(3):201–11.
64. Conboy IM, Conboy MJ, Wagers AJ, et al. Rejuvenation of aged progenitor cells
    by exposure to a young systemic environment. Nature 2005;433(7027):760–4.
65. Rivard A, Berthou-Soulie L, Principe N, et al. Age-dependent defect in vascular
    endothelial growth factor expression is associated with reduced hypoxia-induc-
    ible factor 1 activity. J Biol Chem 2000;275(38):29643–7.
66. Frenkel-Denkberg G, Gershon D, Levy AP. The function of hypoxia-inducible
    factor 1 (HIF-1) is impaired in senescent mice. FEBS Lett 1999;462(3):341–4.

67. Steensma DP, Tefferi A. Anemia in the elderly: how should we define it, when does it matter, and what can be done? Mayo Clin Proc 2007;82(8):958–66.
68. Weiss G, Goodnough LT. Anemia of chronic disease. N Engl J Med 2005;352(10): 1011–23.
69. Greenberg PL, Young NS, Gattermann N. Myelodysplastic syndromes. Hematology Am Soc Hematol Educ Program 2002;136–61.
70. Ferrucci L, Guralnik JM, Woodman RC, et al. Proinflammatory state and circulating erythropoietin in persons with and without anemia. Am J Med 2005; 118(11):1288.
71. Ershler WB, Sheng S, McKelvey J, et al. Serum erythropoietin and aging: a longitudinal analysis. J Am Geriatr Soc 2005;53(8):1360–5.
72. Singh AK, Szczech L, Tang KL, et al. Correction of anemia with epoetin alfa in chronic kidney disease. N Engl J Med 2006;355(20):2085–98.
73. Katodritou E, Verrou E, Hadjiaggelidou C, et al. Erythropoiesis-stimulating agents are associated with reduced survival in patients with multiple myeloma. Am J Hematol 2008;83(9):697–701.
74. Wright JR, Ung YC, Julian JA, et al. Randomized, double-blind, placebo-controlled trial of erythropoietin in non-small-cell lung cancer with disease-related anemia. J Clin Oncol 2007;25(9):1027–32.
75. Mima T, Nishimoto N. Clinical value of blocking IL-6 receptor. Curr Opin Rheumatol 2009;21(3):224–30.
76. Yin MJ, Yamamoto Y, Gaynor RB. The anti-inflammatory agents aspirin and salicylate inhibit the activity of I(kappa)B kinase-beta. Nature 1998;396(6706):77–80.
77. Lanas A, Garcia-Rodriguez LA, Arroyo MT, et al. Risk of upper gastrointestinal ulcer bleeding associated with selective cyclo-oxygenase-2 inhibitors, traditional non-aspirin non-steroidal anti-inflammatory drugs, aspirin and combinations. Gut 2006;55(12):1731–8.
78. Fleischman A, Shoelson SE, Bernier R, et al. Salsalate improves glycemia and inflammatory parameters in obese young adults. Diabetes Care 2008;31(2): 289–94.
79. Mielants H, Veys EM, Verbruggen G, et al. Comparison of serum salicylate levels and gastro-intestinal blood loss between salsalate (Disalcid) and other forms of salicylates. Scand J Rheumatol 1981;10(3):169–73.
80. Cesari M, Penninx BW, Pahor M, et al. Inflammatory markers and physical performance in older persons: the InCHIANTI study. J Gerontol A Biol Sci Med Sci 2004;59(3):242–8.
81. Brugnara C. Iron deficiency and erythropoiesis: new diagnostic approaches. Clin Chem 2003;49(10):1573–8.
82. Knovich MA, Storey JA, Coffman LG, et al. Ferritin for the clinician. Blood Rev 2009;23(3):95–104.
83. Levey AS, Bosch JP, Lewis JB, et al. A more accurate method to estimate glomerular filtration rate from serum creatinine: a new prediction equation. Modification of Diet in Renal Disease Study Group. Ann Intern Med 1999;130(6):461–70.

Inflammation and Immune System Alterations in Frailty

Xu Yao, MD[a,b], Huifen Li, PhD[c], Sean X. Leng, MD, PhD[c],*

KEYWORDS

• Frailty • Inflammation • IL-6 • Monocytic gene expression
• T cells

Frailty is an important and common geriatric syndrome. It is characterized as a state of decreased physiologic reserve and increased vulnerability for subsequent morbidity and mortality.[1–3] Frailty is also described as a clinical phenotype in old age with a loss of complexity in resting dynamics involving multiple physiologic systems, manifested by maladaptive response to stressors, leading to a vicious cycle toward functional decline and other serious adverse health outcomes.[2,4] The phenotypic characteristics of frail older adults are now recognized to be a syndrome consisting of 3 or more of the following: weakness (by grip strength), low physical activity, slowed motor performance (by walking speed), exhaustion, and unintentional weight loss.[1] According to the frailty definition developed by a group of investigators at Johns Hopkins University, frailty is a syndrome when these phenotypic characteristics are present. This status independently predicts several serious adverse health outcomes, including acute illness, falls, hospitalization, disability, dependency, and mortality, adjusting for comorbidities.[1,5] This phenotype definition has been favorably evaluated and compared with other proposed frailty criteria and has been validated in several large older-adult cohorts as well as in various clinical and cultural settings.[6–9] Based on this definition, the estimated prevalence of frailty is 7% to 10% among community-dwelling men and women who are 65 years and older and up to one-third of those who are 80 years and older.[1,10] Because of the profound functional, medical, and

Dr Leng is a current recipient of the Paul Beeson Career Development Award in Aging Research funded by the National Institute on Aging and Private Foundations, K23 AG028963.
[a] Divisions of Allergy & Clinical Immunology and Geriatric Medicine & Gerontology, Johns Hopkins University School of Medicine, Baltimore, MD, USA
[b] Division of Clinical Dermatology, Institute of Dermatology and Skin Diseases Hospital, Peking Union Medical College and Chinese Academy of Medical Sciences, 12 Jiangwangmiao Road, Nanjing 210042, China
[c] Division of Geriatric Medicine and Gerontology, Department of Medicine, Johns Hopkins University School of Medicine, John R Burton Pavilion, 5505 Hopkins Bayview Circle, Baltimore, MD 21224, USA
* Corresponding author.
E-mail address: sleng1@jhmi.edu

socioeconomic consequences of the frailty syndrome, it is imperative to advance our understanding of the pathogenesis and physiologic impact of this syndrome and, with this information, to develop interventional strategies.

A large body of the literature, most rapidly accumulated in the past few years, suggests that frail older adults manifest multisystem dysregulation, including that in the musculoskeletal, immune, endocrine, hematologic, and cardiovascular systems, to just name a few.[11,12] This article focuses on frailty-associated inflammation and immune system alterations, which, for the ease of discussion, are categorized as heightened inflammation and alterations in the innate and adaptive immunity (**Fig. 1**). As described later, this heightened inflammatory state seems to play an important role, directly or through its adverse influence on other intermediary pathophysiologic processes, in the pathogenesis of frailty. Importantly, alterations in the innate and adaptive immunity likely also lead to heightened inflammation as well as impairment in vaccine-induced immune protection and increased susceptibility to infections in frail older adults.

THE INNATE IMMUNE SYSTEM AND FRAILTY

The innate immune system is the front line of defense against injury and infection in most living organisms. It provides an immediate response to external stressors and, as such, is critical in the development and shaping of immune responses that, in turn, play a central role in inflammation and immune protection against infections. The major cellular components of the innate immune system include neutrophils, monocytes, and dendritic cells, although multiple other cell types, such as fibroblasts and hepatocytes, are also capable of mounting an inflammatory response to stressors. Emerging evidence from a variety of sources suggests that the innate immune system is altered in frailty. The cellular and molecular data presented below support that the innate immune system is overall more active in the frail than in nonfrail older adults.

Elevated Markers of Inflammation in Frailty

The aging immune system is characterized by a low-grade, chronic, systemic inflammatory state, so-called InflammAging.[13] This inflammatory phenotype is marked by

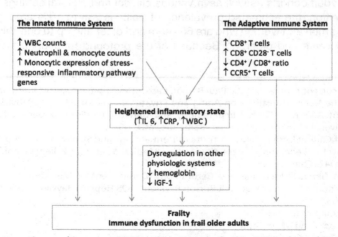

Fig. 1. Inflammation and immune system alterations in frailty. CCR5, chemokine CC receptor 5; CRP, C-reactive protein; IGF-1, insulinlike growth factor 1; IL-6, interleukin 6; WBC, white blood cell.

the presence of elevated inflammatory molecules and is associated with increased morbidity and mortality in older adults.[14,15] C-reactive protein (CRP) and proinflammatory cytokines interleukin (IL)-6 are such well-known inflammatory molecules. Peripheral white blood cell (WBC) and its subpopulations are circulating immune cells and cellular inflammatory components. Clinically, increase in WBC counts is recognized as an important cellular marker of systemic inflammation. Recent studies have provided a large body of evidence that suggests a heightened inflammatory state in frail older adults as marked by further increases in the levels of these molecular and cellular inflammatory markers compared with that observed in nonfrail, robust, older individuals.

IL-6 is a proinflammatory cytokine with increased circulating levels in older adults. Age-related increases in IL-6 levels are associated with several pathophysiologic processes, including atherosclerosis, osteoporosis, and sarcopenia, and with functional decline, disability, and all-cause mortality in older adults.[16-19] In addition, increased IL-6 levels are associated with lower muscle mass and strength even in well-functioning older men and women.[19,20] In a longitudinal study, Ferrucci and colleagues[21] reported that elevated IL-6 levels at baseline predict a significantly higher risk for the development of physical disability and a steeper decline in muscle strength and motor performance during a follow-up period of 3.5 years in older women living in the community. This study and others have shown that chronic systemic inflammation marked by elevated IL-6 levels is associated with decreased muscle strength and power and slowed walking speed, 2 central components of the frailty syndrome. Direct evidence supporting the relationship of this molecular inflammatory marker with frailty came first from a pilot study in which community-dwelling frail older adults had significantly higher levels of IL-6 than nonfrail controls with similar age.[22] A subsequent age-, race-, and sex-matched pair study has further demonstrated that frail older adults had significantly higher IL-6 production by the peripheral blood mononuclear cells (PBMCs), on stimulation with lipopolysaccharide (LPS), than nonfrail controls.[23] In addition, recent studies in large cohorts of older women have demonstrated that elevated IL-6 levels are independently associated with frailty.[24,25] In an IL-10 knockout mouse model for frailty, older mice with phenotype mimicking human frailty had elevated IL-6 levels compared with the control wild type mice.[26] These clinical, laboratory, and population studies have provided strong evidence for the association of this important proinflammatory cytokine with frailty in older adults living in the community.

CRP, discovered in 1930 as an acute phase reactant, is a classic circulating molecular marker of systemic inflammation.[27] Elevated CRP levels are associated with cardiovascular diseases.[28] Clinically, CRP has now been integrated as a part of the routinely measured panel of cardiovascular disease risk factors. The direct association of this molecular inflammatory marker with frailty was demonstrated in 2 large cohort studies. In the Cardiovascular Health Study, Walston and colleagues[29] showed the significant association of elevated CRP levels with frailty after excluding cardiovascular disease and diabetes and adjusting for basic demographic characteristics. Data from the Longitudinal Aging Study Amsterdam have further confirmed these findings.[30]

As part of the complete blood cell counts, WBC count is a standardized and widely available laboratory measurement. Acute and dramatic increase in total WBC counts (above the normal range) is recognized as a clinical indicator for systemic inflammation, frequently because of acute bacterial infections. Several large cohort studies in older adults have demonstrated that elevated WBC count, albeit within the normal range, is associated with cardiovascular and cerebrovascular events, cardiovascular and cancer mortality, as well as all-cause mortality in older adults.[31–33] Recent studies have demonstrated direct relationship of frailty with elevated counts of WBC as well as of neutrophils and monocytes.[24,34] A potential synergistic interaction between WBC and IL-6 in their associations with frailty has also been suggested.[24] The potential synergy between these two commonly recognized cellular and molecular inflammatory components in frailty is further supported by the laboratory study cited earlier in which the PBMCs, the isolated WBC subpopulations, from frail older adults had significantly higher LPS-induced IL-6 production than that from matched nonfrail controls.[23] In addition, direct in vivo association between circulating IL-6 levels and WBC counts has been demonstrated in the same study cohort.[35]

Molecular Inflammatory Pathway Activation in Frailty

Molecular evidence for inflammatory pathway activation in frailty has recently emerged through in-depth analyses of ex vivo expression of inflammatory pathway genes by purified monocytes.[36,37] Using molecular and genetic techniques, including pathway-specific gene array analysis and quantitative real-time reverse-transcriptase polymerase chain reaction, these studies have shown frailty-associated upregulation in the monocytic expression of CXCL10 gene that encodes a potent proinflammatory chemokine.[36] Moreover, purified monocytes from frail older adults had consistent upregulation in ex vivo expression of 7 stress-responsive inflammatory pathway genes on LPS stimulation compared with those from matched nonfrail older adult controls.[37] These genes encode transcription factors, signal transduction proteins, as well as chemokines and cytokines. Findings from these in-depth molecular analyses have demonstrated frailty-associated upregulation in the expression of specific inflammatory pathway genes by monocytes, a major cell type of the innate immune system. As a potential underlying molecular and immune mechanism, upregulated expression of these inflammatory pathway genes could lead to a heightened inflammatory state in frail older adults. This possibility is further suggested by the correlation between frailty-associated CXCL10 upregulation and elevation of serum IL-6 levels, albeit the directionality of this association remains to be determined.[36] In addition, frailty-associated upregulation in the monocytic expression of hydrogen peroxide–induced clone 5, a transcription factor that is known to respond to oxidative stress and play an important role in cellular senescence,[38] suggests a mechanistic link of oxidative stress and cellular senescence with frailty. Such mechanistic link can potentially open novel investigational avenues in frailty research. Moreover, the identified inflammatory pathway genes are stress-responsive genes whose products are known to play a role in stress responses in various study settings.[38–42] This finding is consistent with the cardinal feature of frailty that frail elderly people manifest increased vulnerability to stressors. Clinically, frail older adults may experience LPS exposure surges during gram-negative bacterial infections, such as urinary tract infection and urosepsis.

Potential Role of Heightened Inflammation in Frailty

Although the consequences of this chronic activation is unclear, evidence is also emerging that chronic exposure to inflammatory mediators may be in part responsible for a host of tissue changes and susceptibility to the development of chronic disease states. The relationship between frailty and common molecular and cellular inflammatory markers are well documented. The critical question is whether this heightened inflammation plays a role in the pathogenesis of frailty. Individual inflammatory molecules, such as IL-6, may directly contribute to frailty or its central components (such as decreased muscle strength and power and slowed motor performance). In addition, frailty involves multiple physiologic organ systems, such as musculoskeletal system (sarcopenia, osteopenia), hematologic system (anemia), cardiovascular system (clinical or subclinical cardiovascular diseases), and endocrine system (decreased insulinlike growth factor 1 [IGF-1], decreased dehydroepiandrosterone sulfate, and insulin resistance).[11,12,43] It is conceivable that heightened inflammation contributes to frailty through its detrimental effects (functional impairment and/or structural damage) to these physiologic organ systems. In fact, studies have shown that circulating IL-6 levels have inverse associations with hemoglobin concentration and IGF-1 levels in frail older adults, but not in nonfrail controls; low hemoglobin and IGF-1 levels are each independently associated with frailty, as well.[22,43] In addition, WBC counts have an inverse association with IGF-1 levels.[44] Therefore, it is proposed that the heightened inflammatory state plays a key role in the pathogenesis of frailty, directly or through other intermediate pathophysiologic processes.

THE ADAPTIVE IMMUNE SYSTEM AND FRAILTY

Significant remodeling occurs in the adaptive immune system during aging, which includes age-related loss of CD28 expression, skewing immune repertoire to the memory phenotype, T-cell clonal expansion, increased autoimmune antibody production, and altered cytokine expression. This remodeling is considered to be responsible, at least in part, for the inflammatory phenotype or InflammAging, poor immune response to vaccination, and overall immune functional decline observed in older adults. In frailty syndrome, increasing evidence supports significant alterations in the T-cell compartment of the adaptive immune system. The first line of evidence comes from a post hoc analysis of the data from a nested case-control study evaluating the relationship between T-cell subsets and mortality in community-dwelling older women.[45] The results showed that frail older women had significantly higher counts of $CD8^+$ and $CD8^+CD28^-$ T cells than nonfrail older women (n = 24) matched by age and major comorbidities (cancer, arthritis, diabetes, cardiovascular disease, hypertension, and hormone replacement therapy). Although no difference was observed in $CD4^+$ T-cell frequencies between the 2 study groups, the frail group had a significantly lower $CD4^+:CD8^+$ ratio than the nonfrail group.

The second line of evidence comes from studies in the Multicenter AIDS Cohort Study (MACS) on human immunodeficiency virus (HIV)-positive and HIV-negative gay men. In the MACS study cohort, Desquilbet and colleagues[46] developed a frailty-related phenotype (FRP), which includes 4 of the 5 Fried frailty criteria, with measured walking speed being substituted by self-reported difficulty in walking. The results showed that when compared with HIV-uninfected men of similar age, ethnicity, and education, HIV-infected men were more likely to have FRP for all durations of HIV infection ($\leq$ 4, 4.01–8, and 8.01–12 years) before the era of highly active antiretroviral therapies (HAART). In addition, among HIV seroconverters, men who were HIV infected for 4 years or more had FRP prevalence comparable to HIV-uninfected men 10 years older. A subsequent study in the MACS cohort demonstrated that $CD4^+$ T-cell count predicted the development of an FRP among HIV-infected men, independent of HAART use and plasma HIV viral load.[47] These findings suggest a role of $CD4^+$ T-cell dysregulation in the development of frailty in HIV-infected patient population.

In addition, a pilot study in 13 pairs of age-, race-, and sex-matched frail and nonfrail older adults living in the community with a mean age of 84 years (range: 72–94 years) has shown that frail participants had increased counts of T cells expressing chemokine CC receptor 5 (CCR5) compared with the matched nonfrail controls.[48] The increase of $CCR5^+$ T-cell frequencies in the frail elderly cannot be attributed to the frailty-associated CD8$^+$ T-cell expansion because such an increase was also observed in the CD8$^+$ T-cell compartment. In addition, there was a trend toward graded increase in CCR5$^+$ T-cell counts across the frailty scores in the frail participants.[48] CCR5$^+$ T cells have a type-1 proinflammatory phenotype and contribute significantly to several inflammatory conditions.[49,50] Moreover, CCR5 is a well-known coreceptor for type-1 HIV; active development of anti-CCR5–based therapies for HIV infection and AIDS has shown promising results.[51,52] Therefore, findings from this pilot study, if validated, suggest that anti-CCR5–based strategies can potentially be developed for the prevention or delay and treatment of frailty in older adults.

Information about potential B-cell alteration in frailty is extremely limited. Using spectratype analysis of the immunoglobulin complementarity-determining region 3, a recent study evaluated and compared B-cell repertoire diversity between elderly participants from the Swedish NONA Immune Study and young adults.[53] The results showed an age-related decrease in B-cell diversity and a dramatic collapse of the B-cell repertoire in a subset of older individuals who were considered frail. However, details on how frailty was defined in that study were lacking. Ongoing studies indicate that frail older adults have significant impairment in their antibody response to influenza vaccination compared with their nonfrail counterparts (S.X.L., unpublished data, 2010). It is not clear, however, whether this impairment is caused by alterations in the B-cell compartment or secondary to the frailty-associated T-cell dysregulation.

Emerging evidence suggests significant alterations in the adaptive immune system in frailty, particularly in the T-cell compartment, above and beyond age-related immune remodeling. Further investigations into B-cell function and regulation in frailty are needed.

SUMMARY

This article provides an overview of the current understanding of inflammation and immune system alterations in frailty. The immune system alterations observed in frailty are multifaceted, including the heightened inflammation and alterations in the innate and adaptive immune systems. The identified alterations indicate significant immune dysregulation that is likely responsible for the overall immune functional decline and increased susceptibility to infections in the frail older adult population. In addition, these alterations may play an important role in the pathogenesis of frailty. Furthermore, they include molecular targets, such as CXCL10 and CCR5, for the potential development of novel interventional strategies both for the treatment of frailty and for immune functional improvement in the vulnerable elderly population.

ACKNOWLEDGMENTS

We would like to thank members of the Biology of Frailty Program at Johns Hopkins for their input and support. We would also like to thank Denise Baldwin for her excellent secretarial support.

REFERENCES

1. Fried LP, Tangen C, Walston J, et al. Frailty in older adults: evidence for a phenotype. J Gerontol A Biol Sci Med Sci 2001;56A(3):M1–11.
2. Fried LP, Hadley EC, Walston JD, et al. From bedside to bench: research agenda for frailty. Sci Aging Knowledge Environ 2005;2005(31):e24.
3. Walston J, Hadley EC, Ferrucci L, et al. Research agenda for frailty in older adults: toward a better understanding of physiology and etiology: summary

from the American Geriatrics Society/National Institute on Aging Research Conference on Frailty in Older Adults. J Am Geriatr Soc 2006;54(6):991–1001.

4. Lipsitz LA. Dynamics of stability: the physiologic basis of functional health and frailty. J Gerontol A Biol Sci Med Sci 2002;57(3):115–25.

5. Bandeen-Roche K, Xue QL, Ferrucci L, et al. Phenotype of frailty: characterization in the women's health and aging studies. J Gerontol A Biol Sci Med Sci 2006; 61(3):262–6.

6. Rockwood K, Andrew M, Mitnitski A. A comparison of two approaches to measuring frailty in elderly people. J Gerontol A Biol Sci Med Sci 2007;62(7): 738–43.

7. Woods NF, LaCroix AZ, Gray SL, et al. Frailty: emergence and consequences in women aged 65 and older in the women's health initiative observational study. J Am Geriatr Soc 2005;53(8):1321–30.

8. Corapi KM, McGee HM, Barker M. Screening for frailty among seniors in clinical practice. Nat Clin Pract Rheumatol 2006;2(9):476–80.

9. Strandberg TE, Pitkala KH. Frailty in elderly people. Lancet 2007;369(9570): 1328–9.

10. Fried LP, Ferrucci L, Darer J, et al. Untangling the concepts of disability, frailty, and comorbidity: implications for improved targeting and care. J Gerontol A Biol Sci Med Sci 2004;59(3):255–63.

11. Fried LP, Xue QL, Cappola AR, et al. Nonlinear multisystem physiological dysregulation associated with frailty in older women: implications for etiology and treatment. J Gerontol A Biol Sci Med Sci 2009;64(10):1049–57.

12. Leng SX, Tian XP, Qu T. Pathophysiology of frailty: inflammatory, immune, or endocrine? J Gen Med 2008;20:27–32.

13. Franceschi C, Bonafe M, Valensin S, et al. Inflamm-aging. An evolutionary perspective on immunosenescence. Ann N Y Acad Sci 2000;908:244–54.

14. De MM, Franceschi C, Monti D, et al. Inflammation markers predicting frailty and mortality in the elderly. Exp Mol Pathol 2006;80(3):219–27.

15. Roubenoff R, Parise H, Payette HA, et al. Cytokines, insulin-like growth factor 1, sarcopenia, and mortality in very old community-dwelling men and women: the Framingham Heart Study. Am J Med 2003;115(6):429–35.

16. Ershler WB. Interleukin-6: a cytokine for gerontologists. J Am Geriatr Soc 1993; 41(2):176–81.

17. Maggio M, Guralnik JM, Longo DL, et al. Interleukin-6 in aging and chronic disease: a magnificent pathway. J Gerontol A Biol Sci Med Sci 2006;61(6):575–84.

18. Harris TB, Ferrucci L, Tracy RP, et al. Associations of elevated interleukin-6 and C-reactive protein levels with mortality in the elderly. Am J Med 1999;106(5):506–12.

19. Reuben DB, Cheh AI, Harris TB, et al. Peripheral blood markers of inflammation predict mortality and functional decline in high-functioning community-dwelling older persons. J Am Geriatr Soc 2002;50(4):638–44.

20. Visser M, Pahor M, Taaffe DR, et al. Relationship of interleukin-6 and tumor necrosis factor-alpha with muscle mass and muscle strength in elderly men and women: the Health ABC Study. J Gerontol A Biol Sci Med Sci 2002;57(5): M326–32.

21. Ferrucci L, Penninx BW, Volpato S, et al. Change in muscle strength explains accelerated decline of physical function in older women with high interleukin-6 serum levels. J Am Geriatr Soc 2002;50(12):1947–54.

22. Leng S, Chaves P, Koenig K, et al. Serum interleukin-6 and hemoglobin as physiological correlates in the geriatric syndrome of frailty: a pilot study. J Am Geriatr Soc 2002;50(7):1268–71.

23. Leng S, Yang H, Walston J. Decreased cell proliferation and altered cytokine production in frail older adults. Aging Clin Exp Res 2004;16:249–52.
24. Leng SX, Xue QL, Tian J, et al. Inflammation and frailty in older women. J Am Geriatr Soc 2007;55(6):864–71.
25. Schmaltz HN, Fried LP, Xue QL, et al. Chronic cytomegalovirus infection and inflammation are associated with prevalent frailty in community-dwelling older women. J Am Geriatr Soc 2005;53(5):747–54.
26. Walston J, Fedarko N, Yang H, et al. The physical and biological characterization of a frail mouse model. J Gerontol A Biol Sci Med Sci 2008;63(4):391–8.
27. Tillet W, Francis T. Serological reactions in pneumonia with a non-protein somatic fraction of pneumococcus. J Exp Med 1930;52:561–71.
28. Hage FG, Szalai AJ. C-reactive protein gene polymorphisms, C-reactive protein blood levels, and cardiovascular disease risk. J Am Coll Cardiol 2007;50(12): 1115–22.
29. Walston J, McBurnie MA, Newman A, et al. Frailty and activation of the inflammation and coagulation systems with and without clinical morbidities: results from the Cardiovascular Health Study. Arch Intern Med 2002;162:2333–41.
30. Puts MT, Visser M, Twisk JW, et al. Endocrine and inflammatory markers as predictors of frailty. Clin Endocrinol (Oxf) 2005;63(4):403–11.
31. Leng SX, Xue QL, Huang Y, et al. Baseline total and specific differential white blood cell counts and 5-year all-cause mortality in community-dwelling older women. Exp Gerontol 2005;40(12):982–7.
32. Margolis KL, Manson JE, Greenland P, et al. Leukocyte count as a predictor of cardiovascular events and mortality in postmenopausal women: the Women's Health Initiative Observational Study. Arch Intern Med 2005;165(5):500–8.
33. Ruggiero C, Metter EJ, Cherubini A, et al. White blood cell count and mortality in the Baltimore Longitudinal Study of Aging. J Am Coll Cardiol 2007;49(18):1841–50.
34. Leng S, Xue Q, Tian J. Association of neutrophil and monocyte counts with frailty in community-dwelling older women. Exp Gerontol 2009;44:511–6.
35. Leng S, Xue QL, Huang Y, et al. Total and differential white blood cell counts and their associations with circulating interleukin-6 levels in community-dwelling older women. J Gerontol A Biol Sci Med Sci 2005;60(2):195–9.
36. Qu T, Yang H, Walston JD, et al. Upregulated monocytic expression of CXC chemokine ligand 10 (CXCL-10) and its relationship with serum interleukin-6 levels in the syndrome of frailty. Cytokine 2009;46(3):319–24.
37. Qu T, Walston JD, Yang H, et al. Upregulated ex vivo expression of stress-responsive inflammatory pathway genes by LPS-challenged CD14(+) monocytes in frail older adults. Mech Ageing Dev 2009;130(3):161–6.
38. Jia Y, Ransom RF, Shibanuma M, et al. Identification and characterization of hic-5/ARA55 as an hsp27 binding protein. J Biol Chem 2001;276(43):39911–8.
39. Li DP, Periyasamy S, Jones TJ, et al. Heat and chemical shock potentiation of glucocorticoid receptor transactivation requires heat shock factor (HSF) activity modulation of HSF by vanadate and wortmannin. J Biol Chem 2000;275(34): 26058–65.
40. Sasaki T, Wada T, Kishimoto H, et al. The stress kinase mitogen-activated protein kinase kinase (MKK)7 is a negative regulator of antigen receptor and growth factor receptor-induced proliferation in hematopoietic cells. J Exp Med 2001; 194(6):757–68.
41. Barcellos-Hoff MH. How tissues respond to damage at the cellular level: orchestration by transforming growth factor-{beta} (TGF-{beta}). BJR Suppl 2005;27: 123–7.

42. Viswanathan K, Dhabhar FS. Stress-induced enhancement of leukocyte trafficking into sites of surgery or immune activation. Proc Natl Acad Sci U S A 2005;102(16): 5808–13.
43. Leng SX, Cappola AR, Andersen RE, et al. Serum levels of insulin-like growth factor-I (IGF-I) and dehydroepiandrosterone sulfate (DHEA-S), and their relationships with serum interleukin-6, in the geriatric syndrome of frailty. Aging Clin Exp Res 2004 April;16(2):153–7.
44. Leng SX, Hung W, Cappola AR, et al. White blood cell counts, insulin-like growth factor-1 levels, and frailty in community-dwelling older women. J Gerontol A Biol Sci Med Sci 2009;64(4):499–502.
45. Semba RD, Margolick JB, Leng S, et al. T cell subsets and mortality in older community-dwelling women. Exp Gerontol 2005;40(1–2):81–7.
46. Desquilbet L, Jacobson LP, Fried LP, et al. HIV-1 infection is associated with an earlier occurrence of a phenotype related to frailty. J Gerontol A Biol Sci Med Sci 2007;62(11):1279–86.
47. Desquilbet L, Margolick JB, Fried LP, et al. Relationship between a frailty-related phenotype and progressive deterioration of the immune system in HIV-infected men. J Acquir Immune Defic Syndr 2009;50(3):299–306.
48. De FU, Wang GC, Fedarko NS, et al. T-lymphocytes expressing CC chemokine receptor-5 are increased in frail older adults. J Am Geriatr Soc 2008;56(5):904–8.
49. Loetscher P, Uguccioni M, Bordoli L, et al. CCR5 is characteristic of Th1 lymphocytes. Nature 1998;391(6665):344–5.
50. Qin S, Rottman JB, Myers P, et al. The chemokine receptors CXCR3 and CCR5 mark subsets of T cells associated with certain inflammatory reactions. J Clin Invest 1998;101(4):746–54.
51. Liu R, Paxton WA, Choe S, et al. Homozygous defect in HIV-1 coreceptor accounts for resistance of some multiply-exposed individuals to HIV-1 infection. Cell 1996;86(3):367–77.
52. Fatkenheuer G, Pozniak AL, Johnson MA, et al. Efficacy of short-term monotherapy with maraviroc, a new CCR5 antagonist, in patients infected with HIV-1. Nat Med 2005;11(11):1170–2.
53. Gibson KL, Wu YC, Barnett Y, et al. B-cell diversity decreases in old age and is correlated with poor health status. Aging Cell 2009;8(1):18–25.

The Clinical Care of Frail, Older Adults

Fred Chau-Yang Ko, MD

KEYWORDS

- Frailty • Intervention • Exercise • GEM • GCA
- Interdisciplinary care

Frailty and its management represent an emerging area of clinical care in older adults. Geriatricians have long recognized a syndrome of multiple comorbid conditions, immobility, weakness, and poor tolerance of physiologic stressors in older adults.[1] Patients with these characteristics are described as frail and suffer increased adverse clinical outcomes, such as acute illness, falls, disability, institutionalization, and death.[2] Recent advances in research have better characterized frailty syndrome and its pathophysiology, including the dysregulation of homeostasis in musculoskeletal, neuroendocrine, and immune systems. Although curative treatments for frailty are currently unavailable, exercise intervention and geriatric interdisciplinary assessment and treatment models can improve clinical outcomes in this patient population. Given the high morbidity and mortality secondary to frailty, increased awareness of this syndrome, its early diagnosis, and therefore, timely implementation of beneficial interventions are essential in improving health outcomes in affected older adults.

The purpose of this article is to review the clinical spectrum of frailty in older adults, its biologic etiology, and potential clinical interventions. The first section briefly outlines several operational definitions of frailty and the associated clinical signs, symptoms, and outcomes. The second focuses on the biologic mechanisms hypothesized to underlie frailty, particularly in the musculoskeletal, endocrine, and immune systems. The final section discusses treatment options for frail, older adults, including physiologic system-targeted interventions and geriatric models of care. Similar reviews have been published previously.[3–5]

FRAILTY SYNDROME: DEFINITIONS AND CLINICAL OUTCOMES

To provide optimal clinical care for frail older adults, it is pertinent that clinicians recognize the range of signs, symptoms, and adverse outcomes associated with frailty syndrome. Frailty at the end stage is clinically apparent and is often identified through evidence of recurrent falls and injuries, disability, susceptibility to acute illness, and poor ability to recover from acute stress.[6] Although frailty is more common in older

Department of Geriatrics and Palliative Medicine, Mount Sinai School of Medicine, One Gustave L. Levy Place, Box 1070, New York, NY 10029, USA
E-mail address: fred.ko@mssm.edu

Clin Geriatr Med 27 (2011) 89–100
doi:10.1016/j.cger.2010.08.007
0749-0690/11/$ – see front matter © 2011 Elsevier Inc. All rights reserved.

geriatric.theclinics.com

adults and in those with multiple comorbidities, it certainly can occur independent of advanced age, disability, or specific diseases.[2] Various definitions of frailty have been proposed; however, the operational definition of frailty varies widely according to the conceptual framework; none are considered the gold standard, and few, if any, are used in clinical practice.[6] Most definitions of frailty describe a syndrome characterized by progressive multisystem decline, loss of physiologic reserve, and increase vulnerability to disease and death. Although some researchers define frailty by physical parameters, such as decline in muscular strength, mobility, endurance, physical activity, balance, and weight loss,[2,7,8] others view frailty in a broader sense and incorporate cognitive impairment and psychosocial dimensions in its assessment.[3,8,9]

Definitions that use physical decline as a proxy of frailty frequently use instruments that measure performance and functional changes in mobility and strength. For example, Studenski and colleagues[10] demonstrated that lower extremity performance battery of gait speed and chair stand and tandem balance tests were independent quantitative predictors of 12-month hospitalization rate as well as health and functional decline in 487 older adults seen in primary care settings. In the Zutphen Elderly Study, Chin and colleagues[7] compared 3 working definitions of frailty in 450 older men living independently: (1) inactivity plus low energy intake, (2) inactivity plus weight loss, and (3) inactivity plus low body mass index. The combination of inactivity plus weight loss was the most predictive of mortality and functional decline over 3 years of follow-up. Furthermore, men with the combination of inactivity plus weight loss also had overall poorer grip strength and walking speed and increased disability compared with more active men whose weight was stable.

Fried and colleagues[2] conceptualized frailty as a geriatric syndrome resulting from cumulative decline in multiple physiologic systems. Frailty is present when three of 5 criteria (unintentional weight loss, self-reported exhaustion, poor grip strength, slow walking speed, and low physical activity) are present, reflecting the notion that frailty is a syndrome with a critical mass of signs and symptoms and has a stepwise impact on clinical outcomes. The Cardiovascular Health Study (CHS) tested and validated this definition of frailty in 5317 community-dwelling men and women aged 65 years and older. This frailty phenotype was independently predictive of incident falls, worsening mobility or activity of daily living (ADL) disability, hospitalization, and death over 3 years, even after adjusting for health status, socioeconomic status, and disability. The frailty definition developed in the CHS was subsequently validated in a population of community-dwelling older women in the Women's Health and Aging Studies (WHAS).[11]

Other definitions of frailty use clinical information to identify older adults at risk of adverse outcomes.[3] For examples, Rockwood and colleagues[9] included impairment of cognition, mood, mobility, balance, ADLs, instrumental ADLs, nutrition, and other comorbidities in the assessment of frailty. This frailty index has been demonstrated to be highly predictive of mortality and hospitalization in older adults.

BIOLOGIC BASES OF FRAILTY

Although the biologic mechanisms of frailty are not completely understood, its underlying cause is thought to be multisystemic and probably involves the dysregulation of neuromuscular, endocrine, and immune systems.

Skeletal Muscle

Given that weakness and poor physical performance are principal to most definitions of frailty,[12,13] sarcopenia, defined as the loss of muscle mass and strength, is probably a key physiologic contributor to frailty. This process begins after peak muscle mass and strength are attained at ages 20 to 30 years and has an accelerated rate of decline after age 50 years.[14,15] Sarcopenia can be further accelerated by chronic illness and is a major cause of disability and frailty in the elderly.[13] Causes of this physiologic decline include age-related changes in alpha-motor neurons, type I muscle fibers, muscular atrophy, growth hormone (GH) production, sex steroid levels, and physical activity. Also, increased production of catabolic cytokines and poor nutrition are potentially important causes of sarcopenia.[13,16]

Endocrine Systems

Sex steroids and insulinlike growth factor 1 (IGF-1) are central to skeletal muscle metabolism. Changes in regulation of these hormones secondary to aging or disease states are likely to accelerate the decline in muscle strength and mass in older adults with physical frailty.[17] The age-related rapid decrease of estrogen in postmenopausal women and gradual decrease of testosterone in older men lead to decline in muscle mass and muscle strength.[18–20] Serum levels of the sex hormone dehydroepiandrosterone sulfate (DHEA-S) and IGF-1, a signaling target of GH, are significantly lower in frail than nonfrail older women.[21] Furthermore, lower serum IGF-1 level is associated with progressive disability, poor muscle strength, slow walking speed, and increased mortality in the WHAS, suggesting a potential role for GH-IGF-1 somatotropic axis dysregulation in the development of frailty.[22,23]

Several other hormones, including cortisol and vitamin D, have been associated with frailty in older adults. The loss of stringent regulation of the hypothalamic-pituitary-adrenal axis is hypothesized to cause an age-related increase in cortisol production, which leads to decreased skeletal muscle mass and strength.[5] This hypothesis is supported by recent epidemiologic evidence that demonstrates a positive association between higher levels of evening cortisol, 24-hour mean cortisol, and blunted diurnal variation of cortisol, with the frailty burden and clinical presentation observed in frail older women in the WHAS.[24] Finally, low 25-hydroxyvitamin D level, commonly seen in older adults, is a risk factor of falls, fractures, sarcopenia, poor physical function, and disability.[25–27] Recent findings from the prospective cohort Invecchiare (Aging) in Chianti (InCHIANTI) study and the Longitudinal Aging Study Amsterdam (LASA) suggest that vitamin D insufficiency is also associated with prevalent and incident frailty, particularly in older men.[25,26]

Inflammation

Chronic inflammation characterized by chronic elevation of serum levels of proinflammatory cytokine interleukin 6 (IL-6) is strongly associated with frail older adults in the WHAS.[28] Furthermore, C-reactive protein (CRP), an acute-phase reactant directly upregulated by IL-6, is positively associated with baseline and incident frailty in the LASA[25] and CHS.[29] Finally, elevated neutrophils and macrophages are independently associated with prevalent frailty in the WHAS.[30]

Of the known inflammatory changes that occur in frail older adults, high IL-6 is most predictive of poor functional and clinical outcomes in chronic diseases and in frailty. IL-6 is a biologically important cytokine that is tightly regulated by the immune system. Its age-related increase is partially due to the loss of suppression from the decrease in estrogen and testosterone levels that occurs with aging.[31] High and chronically elevated levels of serum IL-6 are strongly associated with multiple disease states (diabetes, anemia, arthrosclerosis, heart failure, and dementia) and predict poor clinical outcomes (increased disability and mortality as well as sarcopenia) in older adults.[31–35] Furthermore, IL-6 may have hematologic effects in frail older adults by activating the clotting cascade (factor VIII, fibrinogen, and D-dimer) and inhibiting erythropoiesis via interference with normal iron metabolism.[29,36] Although the exact mechanism of chronic inflammation in the pathogenesis of frailty remains unknown, the persistent elevation and dysregulation of IL-6 may be a key step in this disease process and a potential target for future interventions.

Multisystemic Contributions to Frailty

The cause of frailty in older adults is likely to be multisystemic rather than due to dys-regulation in a single physiologic system. Although age-related or disease-associated changes in the neuromuscular, endocrine, and inflammatory systems can independently lead to increased vulnerability to poor outcomes in older adults, aggregate alterations in these systems may have synergistic adverse effects. For example, the combination of high IL-6 and low IGF-1 serum levels confers a higher risk of progressive disability and mortality in the cohort of community-dwelling women in the WHAS than either factor alone, suggesting a possible synergistic effect.[21,23] Similarly, greater levels of production of tumor necrosis factor alpha (TNF-α) and IL-6 and decreased IGF-1 are associated with increased mortality in community-dwelling older adults in the Framingham Heart Study.[37] Ultimately, multiple dysregulated systems interacting in nonlinear ways have been shown to be associated with frailty, leading to speculation that interventions in one system may improve other systems.

TREATMENT OPTIONS FOR FRAIL, OLDER ADULTS

To date, exercise and geriatric interdisciplinary assessment and treatment models are the only options that have been demonstrated to improve clinical outcomes in frail, older adults. As understanding of the biologic basis of frailty improves, more effective therapeutic regimens that target specific physiologic systems and alternative models of geriatric care are likely to be developed.

Physiologic-System-Targeted Interventions

Exercise intervention

Aging-related loss of muscle mass and strength due to sarcopenia is a significant cause of disability in frail older adults.[13] Numerous studies have shown that regular exercise training improves muscle strength, aerobic capacity, balance, and mobility and reduces falls in older adults.[38,39] Other benefits of regular exercises include improvement in performance of ADLs, postponement of disability, and continuance of independent living in oldest subjects.[40,41] Also, exercise can reduce chronic elevations in inflammatory mediators.[42]

In a study of frail, female, nursing home residents whose average age was 87 years, Fiatarone and colleagues[43] demonstrated that progressive resistance exercise training resulted in significant increases in muscle strength (113%), gait velocity (12%), and cross-sectional thigh-muscle area (3%), compared with the control group. Stair-climbing power and spontaneous physical activity also increased in the group that participated in exercise intervention, further supporting the idea that high-intensity resistance training could counteract sarcopenia and physical frailty in the very old. Tai Chi, a dynamic balance exercise, was shown to significantly decrease falls in frail, older adults during and after the intervention period in the Frailty and Injuries: Cooperative Studies of Intervention Techniques (FICSIT) trials.[39] Also, meta-analyses of the FICSIT trials showed that exercise significantly improved quality of life and emotional health and that exercise-related joint and muscle stresses did not increase bodily pain in older adults.[44]

In a recent systematic review, Chin and colleagues[38] examined 20 randomized controlled trials published from 1995 to 2007 that evaluated the effects of 23 different exercise training programs on physical performance in older people with varying degrees of frailty. Most of these interventions were facility-based, group-exercise programs composed of resistance training (n = 9); Tai Chi training (n = 2); or multicomponent training, including resistance, endurance, balance, and flexibility exercises (n = 12); performed thrice a week for 45 to 60 minutes. Fourteen of these trials demonstrated a beneficial effect of exercise on functional performance, suggesting that older adults with different levels of baseline functions could benefit from exercise training. Five of the studies that did not show significant benefit of exercise were performed in a highly frail population, suggesting that the degree of frailty may play a role in dictating effectiveness of exercise programs.

In summary, exercise training improves functional performance, fall prevention, quality of life, and emotional health in older, frail patients. Although evidence suggests that a structured exercise program enhances functional performance across the frailty spectrum, its benefits in the most severely frail patients may be limited. Despite these positive outcomes, specific guidelines of exercise programs (type, intensity, frequency, and duration) for frail, older adults have not been established. Because resistance exercise has been shown to be well-tolerated by older adults,[45] resistance training with exercise machines and body weight or elastic bands, with sessions lasting 30 minutes twice a week, should be implemented in frail, older adults who can safely participate. In more frail patients, structured resistance training can be modified and administered with assistance by caretakers for community-dwelling patients or can be incorporated into restorative therapy programs for long-term-care residents.

Hormonal intervention

Because decline in circulating levels of sex steroids, DHEA-S, vitamin D, and IGF-1 are associated with frailty in older adults, hormone replacement may be a potential therapeutic intervention to improve muscle mass and strength and, ultimately, to improve clinical outcomes. However, to date, the efficacy of hormonal replacement therapy in treating frailty has not been established. Hormone therapy is not currently recommended for the clinical management of frail older adults in the absence of clear clinical deficiencies.

Although multiple clinical studies have shown that testosterone replacement in older men can increase lean muscle mass, muscle strength, and aerobic endurance and reduces whole-body and trunk fat, its effect on functional performance has yielded mixed results.[46–49] Because of the absence of consistent beneficial effects of testosterone replacement and its associated adverse effects on prostate enlargement and hyperlipidemia, testosterone replacement as an intervention for frailty is not recommended. Similarly, although vitamin D replacement in older adults with vitamin D deficiency increases muscle strength and function and decreases falls and hip fractures, its efficacy in frailty intervention has not been reported.[19,50,51] Finally, GH administration to older adults with low IGF-1 levels increases lean body mass and bone mineral density and reduces body fat mass, but its effect on frailty remains unknown.[52]

Anti-inflammatory intervention

Although substantial evidence supports the relationship between chronic IL-6 elevation and frailty-related outcomes, including muscle mass decline, disability, and mortality, pharmacologic treatments aimed at reducing inflammation in frail, older adults have not been developed. The use of TNF-α antagonist as an antirheumatic agent has effectively reduced systemic symptoms of rheumatoid arthritis similar to those observed in frailty, including weakness and fatigue.[53] Because inflammation has a significant etiologic role in rheumatoid arthritis and frailty, using specific anti-inflammatory modulators may potentially delay the onset or progression of frailty while reducing symptoms and improving quality of life.

Models of Care for Frail and Vulnerable Older Adults

Comprehensive geriatric interdisciplinary assessment and treatment

Comprehensive geriatric assessment with implementation of an interdisciplinary treatment plan improves the clinical outcome and quality of life of the frail, older adult.[3,5] The overall objectives of this intervention are to improve physical and psychological function, reduce hospitalization and long-term care placement, improve quality of life, and decrease early mortality in older adults.[54] The interdisciplinary assessment and care team usually consists of a geriatrician, a nurse, a social worker, and an occupational or physical therapist. Patient assessment includes data collection via detailed medical history and physical examination and a thorough discussion and synthesis of relevant psychosocial and medical data and environmental resources, followed by the formulation of treatment goals and management plans developed with the direct participation of the patient and caregivers.

Geriatrics-focused interdisciplinary management of older adults can be grouped into 2 models of care: (1) geriatric evaluation and management (GEM), in which the interdisciplinary team actively follows up on the patient and directs medical care, and (2) comprehensive geriatric assessment (CGA), in which the consultative interdisciplinary team makes specific recommendations to the patient's primary care provider rather than directly implementing care.[3,5] In both the GEM and CGA models, interdisciplinary geriatric assessments associated with ongoing follow-up care targeted at vulnerable older adults have demonstrated improved clinical outcomes. For example, a single outpatient CGA coupled with an adherence intervention prevented functional and quality-of-life decline among community-dwelling older persons who had at least one of the 4 following geriatric conditions: falls, urinary incontinence, depressive symptoms, and functional impairment.[55] Similarly, a meta-analysis on 28 controlled trials of 4959 subjects allocated to CGA linked with long-term management showed improved survival and function in older persons.[56] Boult and colleagues,[57] conducted a randomized controlled trial of GEM intervention targeted at older patients at risk of repeated hospitalization and found that participants of GEM were less likely to lose functional ability, experience increased health-related restrictions in their daily activities, or use home health care services during the 12 to 18 months after randomization. Because CGA and GEM are most effective when treatment plans are implemented, monitored, and revised through close follow-up, the active participation of the patient and caregivers in these interventions is essential to its success.[57] Lastly, the importance of a collaborative relationship between the patient and the primary care physician in CGA should not be understated. It has been shown that patient adherence to CGA treatment plans is significantly increased when the patient and the primary care physician concur on recommended geriatric health care.[58,59]

All-inclusive care for the elderly

Because frail, older adults experience more adverse effects of hospitalization, alternative programs that provide modest medical intervention and palliative care in the patients' home or in the outpatient clinic have been developed. The most widely used model of this type is the Program for All-Inclusive Care of the Elderly (PACE). The core features of PACE include targeting nursing home-eligible participants who choose to receive long-term care services in the community, integrating funding and provider financial risk through capitated Medicare and Medicaid reimbursement, delivering integrated service through adult day care centers, and using interdisciplinary teams for case management.[60] The interdisciplinary team consists of trained geriatrics providers, nurses, physical and occupational therapists, and social workers. Additional patient-centered services include home nursing and home health aide services, transportation, and adult day care. The goals of PACE are to improve patients' functional status and to maintain quality of life by allowing frail older adults to remain in their communities and by preventing institutionalization. Patients enrolled in this program receive complete long-term care and are transitioned to appropriate settings of care, including hospitals, assisted living, nursing homes, and palliative care, as clinically indicated. Although initially conceived as a community-based program, variations of the PACE model have recently been successfully demonstrated in 3 Veterans Affairs (VA) medical centers.[61] The successful partnership of PACE with the VA to provide care for veterans suggests that PACE should not be viewed as a niche program and that other VA-community partnerships for care provision of frail older adults should be identified and implemented.

The acute care for elders model

Similar to outpatient management of older adults, the geriatrician-led interdisciplinary team approach has been shown to improve functional status, reduce acute care hospital days and readmission, and lower mortality rate in hospitalized acutely ill frail older patients.[62,63] The most frequently used model to deliver interdisciplinary inpatient care for frail older patients is the Acute Care for Elderly (ACE) unit. Key features of the ACE unit include a more homelike environment, patient-centered care that includes plans for preventing disability and iatrogenic illness, and comprehensive discharge planning and management.[64] In a randomized control trial of older community-dwelling patients admitted to a hospital for acute medical illnesses, ACE intervention decreased ADL decline or nursing home placement and improved provider and patient satisfaction without increasing hospital length of stay or costs.[64]

Screening and Treatment Algorithm

Physicians who are not familiar with the clinical care of frail, older adults may not easily recognize frailty in its early stage. Also, the lack of a uniform definition and diagnostic criteria make early diagnosis of frailty syndrome difficult. Therefore, assessment tools that can predict the risk of functional decline, disability, and frailty and instruments that can be easily administered during routine physician visits by nongeriatricians should be used as screening tools for frailty.[65] Examples of these assessment tools include the physical performance battery of gait speed, standing balance, and time to rise from chair[66]; the Edmonton frail scale[67]; and the validated CHS frailty phenotype.[2]

In managing older adults, diseases such as major depression, heart failure, and occult malignancy with symptoms overlapping those of frailty need to be ruled out and treated first. Once a frail, older adult is identified, the patient should be initiated on exercise intervention and referred for geriatrics-focused interdisciplinary management (GEM, CGA; **Fig. 1**). A patient who is nursing home-eligible should be referred to PACE for all-inclusive care. In an increasingly frail patient, caretakers should implement structured resistance training programs at home or through community resources (adult day care and senior centers with exercise therapy) and long-term care facilities (restorative therapy). In an acutely ill frail older adult, inpatient management should be delivered in an ACE unit. In the frailest patient, palliative care should be considered and implemented if appropriate. Finally, it is crucial that patient-centered

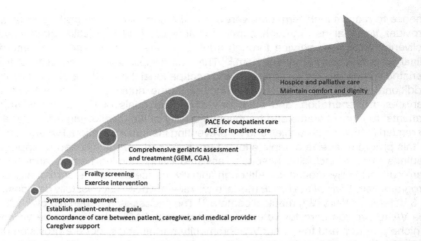

Fig. 1. Clinical management along the spectrum of frailty in older adults. The direction of arrow reflects increasing frailty. Each circle indicates potentially beneficial interventions at different stages of frailty syndrome.

goals remain the focus of the management plan and that the patient, the caregivers, and the interdisciplinary team concur on recommended care throughout the spectrum of frailty in older adults.

SUMMARY

Frailty in older adults is associated with high morbidity and mortality. Clinicians should have heightened awareness of the signs and symptoms of frailty syndrome, make timely diagnosis, and implement exercise therapy and geriatrics-focused interdisciplinary management to improve health outcome in this most vulnerable subset of older adults. Although curative therapy for frailty is not available, advances in frailty research is likely to lead to improved pharmacologic or nonpharmacologic interventions in the near future.

REFERENCES

1. Walston J. Frailty–the search for underlying causes. Sci Aging Knowledge Environ 2004;2004(4):pe4.
2. Fried LP, Tangen CM, Walston J, et al. Frailty in older adults: evidence for a phenotype. J Gerontol A Biol Sci Med Sci 2001;56(3):M146–56.
3. Espinoza S, Walston JD. Frailty in older adults: insights and interventions. Cleve Clin J Med 2005;72(12):1105–12.
4. Morley JE. Developing novel therapeutic approaches to frailty. Curr Pharm Des 2009;15(29):3384–95.
5. Walston JD, Fried LP. Frailty and its implications for care. In: Morrison RS, Meir DE, editors. Geriatric palliative care. New York: Oxford University Press; 2003. p. 93–109.
6. Hamerman D. Toward an understanding of frailty. Ann Intern Med 1999;130(11): 945–50.
7. Chin A, Paw MJ, Dekker JM, et al. How to select a frail elderly population? a comparison of three working definitions. J Clin Epidemiol 1999;52(11):1015–21.

8. Ferrucci L, Guralnik JM, Studenski S, et al. Designing randomized, controlled trials aimed at preventing or delaying functional decline and disability in frail, older persons: a consensus report. J Am Geriatr Soc 2004;52(4):625–34.
9. Rockwood K, Stadnyk K, MacKnight C, et al. A brief clinical instrument to classify frailty in elderly people. Lancet 1999;353(9148):205–6.
10. Studenski S, Perera S, Wallace D, et al. Physical performance measures in the clinical setting. J Am Geriatr Soc 2003;51(3):314–22.
11. Bandeen-Roche K, Xue QL, Ferrucci L, et al. Phenotype of frailty: characterization in the women's health and aging studies. J Gerontol A Biol Sci Med Sci 2006; 61(3):262–6.
12. Evans WJ. What is sarcopenia? J Gerontol A Biol Sci Med Sci 1995;50(Spec No): 5–8.
13. Roubenoff R. Sarcopenia: a major modifiable cause of frailty in the elderly. J Nutr Health Aging 2000;4(3):140–2.
14. Metter EJ, Conwit R, Tobin J, et al. Age-associated loss of power and strength in the upper extremities in women and men. J Gerontol A Biol Sci Med Sci 1997; 52(5):B267–76.
15. Rice CL, Cunningham DA, Paterson DH, et al. Arm and leg composition determined by computed tomography in young and elderly men. Clin Physiol 1989; 9(3):207–20.
16. Larsson L, Ramamurthy B. Aging-related changes in skeletal muscle. mechanisms and interventions. Drugs Aging 2000;17(4):303–16.
17. Morley JE, Baumgartner RN, Roubenoff R, et al. Sarcopenia. J Lab Clin Med 2001;137(4):231–43.
18. Morley JE, Kaiser FE, Sih R, et al. Testosterone and frailty. Clin Geriatr Med 1997; 13(4):685–95.
19. O'Donnell AB, Araujo AB, McKinlay JB. The health of normally aging men: The Massachusetts Male Aging Study (1987–2004). Exp Gerontol 2004;39(7):975–84.
20. Poehlman ET, Toth MJ, Fishman PS, et al. Sarcopenia in aging humans: the impact of menopause and disease. J Gerontol A Biol Sci Med Sci 1995; 50(Spec No):73–7.
21. Leng SX, Cappola AR, Andersen RE, et al. Serum levels of insulin-like growth factor-I (IGF-I) and dehydroepiandrosterone sulfate (DHEA-S), and their relationships with serum interleukin-6, in the geriatric syndrome of frailty. Aging Clin Exp Res 2004;16(2):153–7.
22. Cappola AR, Bandeen-Roche K, Wand GS, et al. Association of IGF-I levels with muscle strength and mobility in older women. J Clin Endocrinol Metab 2001; 86(9):4139–46.
23. Cappola AR, Xue QL, Ferrucci L, et al. Insulin-like growth factor I and interleukin-6 contribute synergistically to disability and mortality in older women. J Clin Endocrinol Metab 2003;88(5):2019–25.
24. Varadhan R, Walston J, Cappola AR, et al. Higher levels and blunted diurnal variation of cortisol in frail older women. J Gerontol A Biol Sci Med Sci 2008; 63(2):190–5.
25. Puts MT, Visser M, Twisk JW, et al. Endocrine and inflammatory markers as predictors of frailty. Clin Endocrinol (Oxf) 2005;63(4):403–11.
26. Shardell M, Hicks GE, Miller RR, et al. Association of low vitamin D levels with the frailty syndrome in men and women. J Gerontol A Biol Sci Med Sci 2009;64(1): 69–75.
27. Visser M, Deeg DJ, Lips P. Low vitamin D and high parathyroid hormone levels as determinants of loss of muscle strength and muscle mass (sarcopenia): the

Longitudinal Aging Study Amsterdam. J Clin Endocrinol Metab 2003;88(12): 5766–72.

28. Leng S, Chaves P, Koenig K, et al. Serum interleukin-6 and hemoglobin as physiological correlates in the geriatric syndrome of frailty: a pilot study. J Am Geriatr Soc 2002;50(7):1268–71.

29. Walston J, McBurnie MA, Newman A, et al. Frailty and activation of the inflammation and coagulation systems with and without clinical comorbidities: results from the cardiovascular health study. Arch Intern Med 2002;162(20):2333–41.

30. Leng SX, Xue QL, Tian J, et al. Inflammation and frailty in older women. J Am Geriatr Soc 2007;55(6):864–71.

31. Ershler WB, Keller ET. Age-associated increased interleukin-6 gene expression, late-life diseases, and frailty. Annu Rev Med 2000;51:245–70.

32. Cesari M, Penninx BW, Newman AB, et al. Inflammatory markers and cardiovascular disease (the health, aging and body composition [health ABC] study). Am J Cardiol 2003;92(5):522–8.

33. Cohen HJ, Harris T, Pieper CF. Coagulation and activation of inflammatory pathways in the development of functional decline and mortality in the elderly. Am J Med 2003;114(3):180–7.

34. Harris TB, Ferrucci L, Tracy RP, et al. Associations of elevated interleukin-6 and C-reactive protein levels with mortality in the elderly. Am J Med 1999;106(5): 506–12.

35. Pradhan AD, Manson JE, Rifai N, et al. C-reactive protein, interleukin 6, and risk of developing type 2 diabetes mellitus. JAMA 2001;286(3):327–34.

36. Ershler WB. Biological interactions of aging and anemia: a focus on cytokines. J Am Geriatr Soc 2003;51(Suppl 3):S18–21.

37. Roubenoff R, Parise H, Payette HA, et al. Cytokines, insulin-like growth factor 1, sarcopenia, and mortality in very old community-dwelling men and women: the Framingham Heart Study. Am J Med 2003;115(6):429–35.

38. Chin A, Paw MJ, van Uffelen JG, et al. The functional effects of physical exercise training in frail older people: a systematic review. Sports Med 2008; 38(9):781–93.

39. Province MA, Hadley EC, Hornbrook MC, et al. The effects of exercise on falls in elderly patients. a preplanned meta-analysis of the FICSIT trials. frailty and injuries: cooperative studies of intervention techniques. JAMA 1995;273(17):1341–7.

40. Keysor JJ. Does late-life physical activity or exercise prevent or minimize disablement? a critical review of the scientific evidence. Am J Prev Med 2003; 25(3 Suppl 2):129–36.

41. Spirduso WW, Cronin DL. Exercise dose-response effects on quality of life and independent living in older adults. Med Sci Sports Exerc 2001;33(6 Suppl): S598–608 [discussion: S609–10].

42. Nicklas BJ, Brinkley TE. Exercise training as a treatment for chronic inflammation in the elderly. Exerc Sport Sci Rev 2009;37(4):165–70.

43. Fiatarone MA, O'Neill EF, Ryan ND, et al. Exercise training and nutritional supplementation for physical frailty in very elderly people. N Engl J Med 1994; 330(25):1769–75.

44. Schechtman KB, Ory MG. Frailty and Injuries: Cooperative Studies of Intervention Techniques. The effects of exercise on the quality of life of frail older adults: a preplanned meta-analysis of the FICSIT trials. Ann Behav Med 2001;23(3): 186–97.

45. Lang T, Streeper T, Cawthon P, et al. Sarcopenia: etiology, clinical consequences, intervention, and assessment. Osteoporos Int 2009;21(4):543–59.

46. Ottenbacher KJ, Ottenbacher ME, Ottenbacher AJ, et al. Androgen treatment and muscle strength in elderly men: a meta-analysis. J Am Geriatr Soc 2006; 54(11):1666–73.

47. Page ST, Amory JK, Bowman FD, et al. Exogenous testosterone (T) alone or with finasteride increases physical performance, grip strength, and lean body mass in older men with low serum T. J Clin Endocrinol Metab 2005; 90(3):1502–10.

48. Sattler FR, Castaneda-Sceppa C, Binder EF, et al. Testosterone and growth hormone improve body composition and muscle performance in older men. J Clin Endocrinol Metab 2009;94(6):1991–2001.

49. Storer TW, Woodhouse L, Magliano L, et al. Changes in muscle mass, muscle strength, and power but not physical function are related to testosterone dose in healthy older men. J Am Geriatr Soc 2008;56(11):1991–9.

50. Bischoff-Ferrari HA, Dawson-Hughes B, Staehelin HB, et al. Fall prevention with supplemental and active forms of vitamin D: a meta-analysis of randomised controlled trials. BMJ 2009;339:b3692.

51. Bischoff-Ferrari HA, Willett WC, Wong JB, et al. Prevention of nonvertebral fractures with oral vitamin D and dose dependency: a meta-analysis of randomized controlled trials. Arch Intern Med 2009;169(6):551–61.

52. Savine R, Sonksen P. Growth hormone - hormone replacement for the somato-pause? Horm Res 2000;53(Suppl 3):37–41.

53. Criscione LG, St Clair EW. Tumor necrosis factor-alpha antagonists for the treatment of rheumatic diseases. Curr Opin Rheumatol 2002;14(3):204–11.

54. Urdangarin CF. Comprehensive geriatric assessment and management. In: Kane RL, Kane RA, editors. Assessing older person. New York: Oxford University Press; 2000. p. 383–405.

55. Reuben DB, Frank JC, Hirsch SH, et al. A randomized clinical trial of outpatient comprehensive geriatric assessment coupled with an intervention to increase adherence to recommendations. J Am Geriatr Soc 1999;47(3):269–76.

56. Stuck AE, Siu AL, Wieland GD, et al. Comprehensive geriatric assessment: a meta-analysis of controlled trials. Lancet 1993;342(8878):1032–6.

57. Boult C, Boult LB, Morishita L, et al. A randomized clinical trial of outpatient geriatric evaluation and management. J Am Geriatr Soc 2001;49(4):351–9.

58. Maly RC, Leake B, Frank JC, et al. Implementation of consultative geriatric recommendations: the role of patient-primary care physician concordance. J Am Geriatr Soc 2002;50(8):1372–80.

59. Shah PN, Maly RC, Frank JC, et al. Managing geriatric syndromes: what geriatric assessment teams recommend, what primary care physicians implement, what patients adhere to. J Am Geriatr Soc 1997;45(4):413–9.

60. Eng C, Pedulla J, Eleazer GP, et al. Program of all-inclusive care for the elderly (PACE): an innovative model of integrated geriatric care and financing. J Am Geriatr Soc 1997;45(2):223–32.

61. Weaver FM, Hickey EC, Hughes SL, et al. Providing all-inclusive care for frail elderly veterans: evaluation of three models of care. J Am Geriatr Soc 2008; 56(2):345–53.

62. Landefeld CS, Palmer RM, Kresevic DM, et al. A randomized trial of care in a hospital medical unit especially designed to improve the functional outcomes of acutely ill older patients. N Engl J Med 1995;332(20):1338–44.

63. Rubenstein LZ, Josephson KR, Wieland GD, et al. Effectiveness of a geriatric evaluation unit. a randomized clinical trial. N Engl J Med 1984;311(26): 1664–70.

64. Counsell SR, Holder CM, Liebenauer LL, et al. Effects of a multicomponent intervention on functional outcomes and process of care in hospitalized older patients: a randomized controlled trial of acute care for elders (ACE) in a community hospital. J Am Geriatr Soc 2000;48(12):1572–81.
65. Corapi KM, McGee HM, Barker M. Screening for frailty among seniors in clinical practice. Nat Clin Pract Rheumatol 2006;2(9):476–80.
66. Guarente L, Kenyon C. Genetic pathways that regulate ageing in model organisms. Nature 2000;408(6809):255–62.
67. Rolfson DB, Majumdar SR, Tsuyuki RT, et al. Validity and reliability of the Edmonton Frail Scale. Age Ageing 2006;35(5):526–9.

Exercise as an Intervention for Frailty

Christine K. Liu, MD[a,b], Roger A. Fielding, PhD[b],*

KEYWORDS

• Exercise • Frailty • Elderly • Older adults

By 2015, nearly 15% of the US population will be older than 65 years. In 2030, there will be more than 70 million older Americans.[1] This increase in the elderly population has prompted interest in recent years toward the study of frail older adults. Clinicians use the term frail to describe a person older than 65 years who is vulnerable to any kind of change in health status, such as infection or physical injury.[2] These individuals are at a high risk for complications during a medical illness and have prolonged recovery times.[3] An international consensus report in 2006 characterized frail elders as having impairments in mobility, balance, strength, motor processing, cognition, nutrition, endurance (fatigue), and physical activity.[4]

In 1992, Buchner and Wagner[5] first proposed a formal definition of frailty as a syndrome of weakness, impaired mobility, balance, and minimal reserve. Using epidemiologic data from the Cardiovascular Health Study (CHS), Fried and colleagues[2] further characterized individuals with frailty as those who had unintentional weight loss (4.5 kg or more in the past year), fatigue or exercise intolerance, weakness, slowed motor performance, and low physical activity. A person was considered frail if they demonstrated at least 3 of these attributes (**Fig. 1**) and prefrail if they had 1 or 2 of these characteristics. Fried and colleagues[2] found that those who were frail had an increased risk of falls, activities of daily living (ADL) disability, hospitalization, and death over a 3-year period. In the Women's Health and Aging I study, the risk of ADL dependence increased with the number of frailty criteria fulfilled.[6] At

Dr Liu was supported by a Health Resources and Services Administration grant from the Bureau of Health Professions (# D01 HP08796) and by Boston Medical Center, Boston, MA. Dr Fielding was supported by the Boston Claude D. Pepper Older Americans Independence Center (1P30AG031679). This material is based on work supported by the US Department of Agriculture, under agreement No. 58–1950–7–707.
[a] Section of Geriatrics, Department of Medicine, Boston University School of Medicine, 88 East Newton Street, Boston, MA 02118, USA
[b] Nutrition, Exercise Physiology and Sarcopenia Laboratory, Jean Mayer USDA Human Nutrition Research Center on Aging, Tufts University, 711 Washington Street, Boston, MA 02111, USA
* Corresponding author.
E-mail address: roger.fielding@tufts.edu

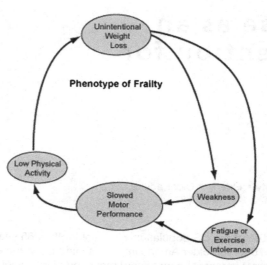

Fig. 1. Components of frailty. (*Adapted from* Fried LP, Xue QL, Cappola AR, et al. Nonlinear multisystem physiologic dysregulation associated with frailty in older women: implications for etiology and treatment. J Gerontol A Biol Sci Med Sci 2009;64(10):1050; with permission.)

7 years, mortality in the frail cohort of the CHS was approximately 3 times higher when compared with the nonfrail cohort (43% vs 12%). About 25% of frail subjects in the CHS had only one chronic disease, defined as osteoarthritis, diabetes, hypertension, angina, congestive heart failure, cancer, or pulmonary disease,[2] suggesting that frailty was not always associated with multiple comorbidities. The underlying mechanisms causing the phenotype of frailty remain to be fully elucidated. Buchner and Wagner[5] initially proposed that declines in neurologic processes, musculoskeletal functioning, and energy metabolism were the causes of frailty. Lipsitz[7] later suggested that frailty might be caused by the loss of the ability of the cardiovascular and nervous systems to respond appropriately to stressors caused by age-related changes. Using these concepts, frailty is now thought to be caused by altered function in multiple physiologic systems (including inflammatory, skeletal muscle, endocrine, clotting, and hematologic) and dysregulation of mechanisms between these systems to maintain homeostasis.[8]

With increasing age, there is a well-described decline in voluntary physical activity, which is associated with decreases in several measures of exercise tolerance, including maximal aerobic capacity, muscle strength, and fatigability,[9] leading to an increased risk of frailty. In recent years, increased physical activity or regular exercise training has been proposed as a preventive strategy for frailty and its adverse outcomes because it can target 4 of the frailty criteria: weakness, low physical activity, slowed motor performance, and exercise intolerance. Epidemiologic studies suggest that regular physical activity is associated with a decreased risk of ADL disability in older adults, which is an adverse outcome of frailty. In a large-scale cohort study in Taiwan, Wu and colleagues[10] found that older adults who were physically active, defined as participating in dancing, hiking, jogging, or walking at least twice a week, were less likely to have ADL disabilities at the end of a 3-year period when compared with their sedentary counterparts. These findings were confirmed by the Longitudinal Study of Aging, which found elders who were physically active, defined as walking at least a mile a week, were less likely to develop impairments in their ADL or instrumental ADLs over a 6-year period, after adjusting for age, gender, comorbidities, and baseline disability.[11]

This article reviews the literature investigating the utility of aerobic and resistance exercise training as an intervention for frailty in older adults. In addition, areas of future research are addressed, including concerns related to the dissemination of exercise interventions on a widespread scale. Also, guidelines for an "exercise prescription" for frail older adults are briefly outlined.

AEROBIC OR ENDURANCE EXERCISE TRAINING

There are 2 mechanisms by which aerobic exercise is thought to alter the frailty phenotype: improvement in the maximal oxygen uptake (Vo_2max) and increased muscle mass. Vo_2max is defined as the maximum rate of oxygen consumption measured during vigorous exercise and is closely related to submaximal endurance exercise capacity and exercise tolerance.

In an intervention study of 64 frail men and women, a 9-month program of strength training and walking that aimed at reaching 78% of peak heart rate, found an increase in endurance by improving Vo_2max by 14%.[12] A small study of healthy, elderly, sedentary women also found that a 12-week regimen of cycle ergometer training improved maximal aerobic capacity by 30% from baseline. This study demonstrated that endurance training increased quadriceps muscle mass by 12%.[13] Although previous studies have shown that aerobic exercise did not alter muscle size in older adults,[14–16] a recent cross-sectional study by Sugawara and colleagues[17] demonstrated that those who undergo aerobic training have a higher percentage of muscle mass in their extremities when compared with their sedentary counterparts.

RESISTANCE EXERCISE TRAINING

There is well-documented evidence that muscle strength decreases with advancing age. Muscle strength decreases approximately 12% to 15% per decade after the age of 50 years[18] in both men and women.[19] In addition, muscle mass also decreases with increased age. In a cross-sectional study of healthy men of equal mass, muscle mass comprised 24% of total mass in those aged 20 to 29 years but decreased to 13% in subjects aged 70 to 79 years.[20] Several studies have found that the decline in strength in older adults is associated with this age-related loss of muscle mass.[21–23] Although resistance exercise training has been shown to increase muscle mass and therefore muscle strength, this response is attenuated in older adults with mobility limitations or other comorbidities. In healthy older men and women, 4 months of resistance training resulted in a 16% to 23% increase in muscle mass compared with a 2.5% to 9% increase in frail or institutionalized older adults.[24–26]

Despite these age-related changes in muscle, resistance exercise training has been found to increase strength in older adults. Multiple studies have demonstrated that these changes can occur even into the ninth decade of life.[24,27–31] In a systemic review of 41 articles by Latham and colleagues,[32] resistance exercise training in older adults was associated with gains in strength, and a Cochrane review of 74 studies found similar results.[33] Both reviews used studies that examined both healthy older adults and frail adults. Fiatarone and colleagues[25] showed that nursing home residents were able to increase their strength on an average of 97% after 10 weeks of resistance exercise training. Because nursing home residents represent the frailest segment of older adults, this study demonstrates that the intervention is beneficial for even those most severely affected by frailty.

Motor performance in older adults has also been shown to improve after resistance training. In their systemic review, Latham and colleagues[32] found that resistance exercise training in healthy and frail elders improved gait speed in 14 studies and increased distance covered in the 6-minute walk test in 6 trials. In their respective studies of frail elders living in the nursing home and in the community, Fiatarone and colleagues[25] and Chandler and colleagues[34] showed that 10 weeks of resistance training resulted in improved gait speed. There may be a dose-response relationship between resistance exercise and motor performance, because Galvao and Taaffe[35] found that subjects who did more repetitions of resistance exercise had almost twice the improvement in their 400-m walk time compared with those who did fewer repetitions.

COMBINED AEROBIC AND RESISTANCE EXERCISE

Given that aerobic or resistance exercise alone has beneficial results and that both types of exercise target specific distinct features of frailty, there has been recent interest in whether an intervention with both components is beneficial for frail older adults. In a randomized controlled trial of elderly subjects who had undergone surgical repair of a femur fracture, a 6-month intervention of aerobic activity and progressive resistance exercise was associated with a mean improvement of 19 m/min in walking speed.[36] Similar changes in motor function were demonstrated in the Lifestyles Interventions and Independence for Elders (LIFE) study, which found that a 12-month program of walking, resistance exercise, and flexibility training improved scores on the Short Physical Performance Battery test and prevented a decline in the 400-m walk speed in older adults at high risk for disability 1 year after follow-up.[37]

EFFECT OF EXERCISE INTERVENTIONS ON THE ADVERSE OUTCOMES OF FRAILTY

Several studies have examined the effect of exercise on reducing the risk of falls, a common adverse outcome of frailty. After a single fall, the risk of skilled nursing facility placement in older adults increases 3-fold, after adjustment for cognitive, psychological, social, functional, and medical factors.[38] In a study examining women undergoing resistance training for 25 weeks, risk of falls was reduced by 57% from baseline.[39] A meta-analysis of 6 studies by Baker and colleagues[40] showed that a combined regimen of aerobic, resistance, balance, and flexibility exercises was found to decrease fall risk. A Cochrane review of 111 trials found that a combination of aerobic and resistance exercise reduced the risk of falls by 17% in community-dwelling elders.[41]

In addition to falls, ADL disability is of major concern in frail individuals because it is associated with higher rates of mortality.[42] In the systemic review of 41 studies conducted by Latham and colleagues,[32] resistance exercise training did not decrease the risk of ADL disability in an elderly population. In contrast, a Cochrane review of 121 trials found an association between resistance training and reduced ADL disability.[33] Neither review stratified their results by the severity of frailty. In a randomized controlled trial of a 6-month home-based program that combined resistance exercise training with balance training and home safety and assistive device evaluations, rates of ADL disability decreased only in those with moderate frailty but not in those with severe frailty. Moderate frailty was defined as the inability to either perform a rapid gait test (requiring >10 seconds to walk a 3-m course) or stand up from a chair with arms folded, and severe frailty was defined as having both characteristics.[43,44] In contrast, Binder and colleagues[45] did not find an improvement in the Older American Resources and Services ADL score in a group of mild to moderately frail subjects after a regimen of resistance, balance, and flexibility training. At present, final results of the

FRASI (FRAilty, Screening and Intervention) are pending;the study observes the effect of an 8-week exercise regimen on the time of onset of ADL disability in community-dwelling frail elders.[46] **Table 1** lists key randomized controlled trials that studied frail older adults.

EFFECT ON THE PHENOTYPE OF FRAILTY

Although there have been multiple trials studying the effects of exercise on the various characteristics of frailty and the adverse outcomes of frailty, there have been few studies to determine whether exercise can alter or even reverse frailty status in older adults. In a study conducted with subjects who were frail or at high risk for frailty, a telephone intervention encouraging exercise decreased the proportion of frail elders by 18% at 6 months follow-up.[47] At present, the Frailty Intervention Trial is examining whether a 12-month intervention of aerobic and resistance training can change frailty status in a cohort of already frail older adults.[48]

ADVERSE OUTCOMES OF EXERCISE

Adverse outcomes with both aerobic and resistance training, although not uncommon, are rarely life threatening. In a study that examined resistance training in elderly women, most of the adverse outcomes were musculoskeletal complaints.[39] Latham and colleagues[49] found that the risk ratio for adverse events increased to 3.6 in those who underwent 10 weeks of resistance training. However, no reports of death or cardiovascular events were found in a systemic review of 62 trials of resistance exercise.[32] In a randomized controlled trial studying the effect of a 12-month intervention of walking, resistance exercise, and flexibility, similar rates of serious and nonserious adverse events were found for both the intervention and control subjects.[37]

FUTURE DIRECTIONS

Clearly, exercise and physical activity are promising interventions for frailty, and several studies are underway to examine their effect. However, there are several related areas that need further investigation before this intervention can be disseminated to frail older adults on a widespread basis. First, adherence to an exercise regimen is key to its beneficial effects, and strategies to overcome this barrier need to be developed before exercise as treatment modality is implemented on a wide scale. Schneider and colleagues[50] found that subjects were interested in exercise for its medical and psychological benefits but had concerns about the time required and their ability to perform adequate exercise. In addition, cognition is a factor that should be considered. A significant proportion of older adults are cognitively impaired, which may affect their ability to properly adhere to a regular exercise regimen. However, if caregivers are involved, cognitive impairment may not be such a barrier. In a randomized clinical trial, subjects with Alzheimer dementia participated in a home-based exercise program of aerobic and resistance exercise under the supervision of their caregivers. At 3 months, the subjects with dementia were more active and had better motor functioning compared with the controls.[51] Almost all the trials reviewed in this article were clinic or facility based. Home-based programs are more accessible and eliminate the barrier of transportation for many elders. In a study that examined a 6-month home-based program that combined resistance and balance training with home safety and assistive device evaluations, there was no improvement in motor performance. However, a later Cochrane review did find that home-based exercise programs reduced the risk of falls in older adults by 23%.[41]

Table 1
Randomized controlled trials in frail older adults

Study	Population	Intervention	Outcome
Fiatarone et al,[25] 1994	Nursing home residents 70 y or older and able to walk 6 m	3 sessions per wk of resistance training of lower extremities for 10 wk vs regular recreational activities	Mean improvement in muscle strength of lower extremities was 97% for intervention group compared with 12% for control group
Chandler et al,[34] 1998	Community-dwelling adults 65 y and older and unable to climb stairs without a handrail	3 sessions per wk of progressive resistance training of lower extremities with stair stepping and chair rises for 10 wk vs normal activities	Mean improvement in muscle strength of lower extremities was 10%–13% for intervention group compared with 1% improvement to 3% decline in control group
Binder et al,[45] 2002	Community-dwelling adults 78 y and older who had 2 of the following criteria: modified PPT score 18–32, Vo₂max 10–18 mL/kg/min, or difficulty with either 1 ADL or 2 IADLs	3 sessions per wk of resistance training of upper and lower extremities; aerobic training with walking, cycling, or rowing; and flexibility/balance training for 9 mo vs flexibility exercises	Mean improvement in lower extremity strength was 19%–23% for intervention group compared with 5% improvement to 5% decline in control group. Mean Vo₂max improved 13% for intervention group compared with 2.6% decline in control group
Gill et al,[44] 2002	Community-dwelling adults 75 y and older who required more than 10 s to walk 3 m and/or unable to stand up from a chair with arms folded	Average of 16 sessions in the home of resistance training of upper and lower extremities, flexibility and balance exercises, and home safety and assistive device evaluations for 6 mo vs education program	66% improvement in disability scores for those with moderate frailty but no significant improvement for those with severe frailty in intervention group, using control group as baseline

Abbreviations: IADLs, instrumental activities of daily living; PPT, Physical Performance Test.

Also, whether these exercise interventions would require supervision by a rehabilitation professional or could be conducted in the community is still unclear. If supervision is necessary, this adds to the cost of the intervention. Future and ongoing trials should include an analysis of the costs and benefits of a physical activity intervention.

SUMMARY: AN EXERCISE "PRESCRIPTION"

Although more investigation is still needed, most studies suggest that clinicians should recommend regular physical activity or exercise training to frail older adults. The current guidelines from the US Department of Health and Human Services state that all adults older than 65 years should participate in 150 minutes (ie, 2.5 hours) of moderate aerobic exercise per week.[52] Although most trials studied resistance exercise training, frail older adults are encouraged to start with an aerobic activity, such as walking, as it is more accessible. If possible, resistance exercise training should be added. Depending on the degree of frailty, supervision may or may not be required. For individuals with severe frailty, evaluation by a rehabilitation professional is recommended.

Most evidence shows that regular physical activity or exercise is beneficial for older adults who are frail or at high risk of frailty. Studies have shown that the number of adverse events is minimal and the gains of regular exercise clearly outweigh the risks. Although there are still several areas related to the intervention that require further investigation, regular physical activity or exercise is highly recommended for older adults as a means to modify frailty and its adverse outcomes.

REFERENCES

1. Available at: www.americangeriatrics.org. Accessed January 14, 2010.
2. Fried LP, Tangen CM, Walston J, et al. Frailty in older adults: evidence for a phenotype. J Gerontol A Biol Sci Med Sci 2001;56(3):M146–56.
3. Fried LP, Ferrucci L, Darer J, et al. Untangling the concepts of disability, frailty, and comorbidity: implications for improved targeting and care. J Gerontol A Biol Sci Med Sci 2004;59(3):255–63.
4. Ferrucci L, Guralnik JM, Studenski S, et al. Designing randomized, controlled trials aimed at preventing or delaying functional decline and disability in frail, older persons: a consensus report. J Am Geriatr Soc 2004;52(4):625–34.
5. Buchner DM, Wagner EH. Preventing frail health. Clin Geriatr Med 1992;8(1): 1–17.
6. Boyd CM, Xue QL, Simpson CF, et al. Frailty, hospitalization, and progression of disability in a cohort of disabled older women. Am J Med 2005;118(11):1225–31.
7. Lipsitz LA. Dynamics of stability: the physiologic basis of functional health and frailty. J Gerontol A Biol Sci Med Sci 2002;57(3):B115–25.
8. Fried LP, Xue QL, Cappola AR, et al. Nonlinear multisystem physiological dysregulation associated with frailty in older women: implications for etiology and treatment. J Gerontol A Biol Sci Med Sci 2009;64(10):1049–57.
9. Walston J, Hadley EC, Ferrucci L, et al. Research agenda for frailty in older adults: toward a better understanding of physiology and etiology: summary from the American Geriatrics Society/National Institute on Aging Research Conference on Frailty in Older Adults. J Am Geriatr Soc 2006;54(6):991–1001.
10. Wu SC, Leu SY, Li CY. Incidence of and predictors for chronic disability in activities of daily living among older people in Taiwan. J Am Geriatr Soc 1999;47(9): 1082–6.

11. Miller ME, Rejeski WJ, Reboussin BA, et al. Physical activity, functional limitations, and disability in older adults. J Am Geriatr Soc 2000;48(10):1264–72.
12. Ehsani AA, Spina RJ, Peterson LR, et al. Attenuation of cardiovascular adaptations to exercise in frail octogenarians. J Appl Physiol 2003;95(5):1781–8.
13. Harber MP, Konopka AR, Douglass MD, et al. Aerobic exercise training improves whole muscle and single myofiber size and function in older women. Am J Physiol Regul Integr Comp Physiol 2009;297(5):R1452–9.
14. Verney J, Kadi F, Saafi MA, et al. Combined lower body endurance and upper body resistance training improves performance and health parameters in healthy active elderly. Eur J Appl Physiol 2006;97(3):288–97.
15. Short KR, Vittone JL, Bigelow ML, et al. Age and aerobic exercise training effects on whole body and muscle protein metabolism. Am J Physiol Endocrinol Metab 2004;286(1):e92–101.
16. Ferrara CM, Goldberg AP, Ortmeyer HK, et al. Effects of aerobic and resistive exercise training on glucose disposal and skeletal muscle metabolism in older men. J Gerontol A Biol Sci Med Sci 2006;61(5):480–7.
17. Sugawara J, Miyachi M, Moreau KL, et al. Age-related reductions in appendicular skeletal muscle mass: association with habitual aerobic exercise status. Clin Physiol Funct Imaging 2002;22(3):169–72.
18. Larsson L. Histochemical characteristics of human skeletal muscle during aging. Acta Physiol Scand 1983;117(3):469–71.
19. Lindle RS, Metter EJ, Lynch NA, et al. Age and gender comparisons of muscle strength in 654 women and men aged 20–93 yr. J Appl Physiol 1997;83(5):1581–7.
20. Munro HN. Aging. In: Kinney JM, Jeejeebhoy KN, Hill GL, et al, editors. Nutrition and metabolism in patient care. Philadelphia: WB Saunders Company; 1988. p. 145–66.
21. Pearson MB, Bassey EJ, Bendall MJ. The effects of age on muscle strength and anthropometric indices within a group of elderly men and women. Age Ageing 1985;14(4):230–4.
22. Frontera WR, Hughes VA, Lutz KJ, et al. A cross-sectional study of muscle strength and mass in 45- to 78-yr-old men and women. J Appl Physiol 1991;71(2):644–50.
23. Newman AB, Haggerty CL, Goodpaster B, et al. Strength and muscle quality in a well-functioning cohort of older adults: the Health, Aging and Body Composition Study. J Am Geriatr Soc 2003;51(3):323–30.
24. Fiatarone MA, Marks EC, Ryan ND, et al. High-intensity strength training in nonagenarians. Effects on skeletal muscle. JAMA 1990;263(22):3029–34.
25. Fiatarone MA, O'Neill EF, Ryan ND, et al. Exercise training and nutritional supplementation for physical frailty in very elderly people. N Engl J Med 1994;330(25):1769–75.
26. Binder EF, Yarasheski KE, Steger-May K, et al. Effects of progressive resistance training on body composition in frail older adults: results of a randomized, controlled trial. J Gerontol A Biol Sci Med Sci 2005;60(11):1425–31.
27. McCartney N, Hicks AL, Martin J, et al. Long-term resistance training in the elderly: effects on dynamic strength, exercise capacity, muscle, and bone. J Gerontol A Biol Sci Med Sci 1995;50(2):B97–104.
28. McCartney N, Hicks AL, Martin J, et al. A longitudinal trial of weight training in the elderly: continued improvements in year 2. J Gerontol A Biol Sci Med Sci 1996;51(6):B425–33.
29. Valkeinen H, Hakkinen K, Pakarinen A, et al. Muscle hypertrophy, strength development, and serum hormones during strength training in elderly women with fibromyalgia. Scand J Rheumatol 2005;34(4):309–14.

30. Ferri A, Scaglioni G, Pousson M, et al. Strength and power changes of the human plantar flexors and knee extensors in response to resistance training in old age. Acta Physiol Scand 2003;177(1):69–78.
31. Adams KJ, Swank AM, Berning JM, et al. Progressive strength training in sedentary, older African American women. Med Sci Sports Exerc 2001;33(9): 1567–76.
32. Latham NK, Bennett DA, Stretton CM, et al. Systematic review of progressive resistance strength training in older adults. J Gerontol A Biol Sci Med Sci 2004;59(1):48–61.
33. Liu CJ, Latham NK. Progressive resistance strength training for improving physical function in older adults. Cochrane Database Syst Rev 2009;3: CD002759.
34. Chandler JM, Duncan PW, Kochersberger G, et al. Is lower extremity strength gain associated with improvement in physical performance and disability in frail, community-dwelling elders? Arch Phys Med Rehabil 1998;79(1):24–30.
35. Galvao DA, Taaffe DR. Resistance exercise dosage in older adults: single- versus multiset effects on physical performance and body composition. J Am Geriatr Soc 2005;53(12):2090–7.
36. Binder EF, Brown M, Sinacore DR, et al. Effects of extended outpatient rehabilitation after hip fracture: a randomized controlled trial. JAMA 2004;292(7):837–46.
37. Pahor M, Blair SN, Espeland M, et al. Effects of a physical activity intervention on measures of physical performance: Results of the Lifestyle Interventions and Independence for Elders Pilot (LIFE-P) study. J Gerontol A Biol Sci Med Sci 2006;61(11):1157–65.
38. Tinetti ME, Williams CS. Falls, injuries due to falls, and the risk of admission to a nursing home. N Engl J Med 1997;337(18):1279–84.
39. Liu-Ambrose T, Khan KM, Eng JJ, et al. Resistance and agility training reduce fall risk in women aged 75 to 85 with low bone mass: a 6-month randomized, controlled trial. J Am Geriatr Soc 2004;52(5):657–65.
40. Baker MK, Atlantis E, Fiatarone Singh MA. Multi-modal exercise programs for older adults. Age Ageing 2007;36(4):375–81.
41. Gillespie LD, Robertson MC, Gillespie WJ, et al. Interventions for preventing falls in older people living in the community. Cochrane Database Syst Rev 2009;2: CD007146.
42. Fried LP, Kronmal RA, Newman AB, et al. Risk factors for 5-year mortality in older adults: the Cardiovascular Health Study. JAMA 1998;279(8):585–92.
43. Gill TM, Baker DI, Gottschalk M, et al. A prehabilitation program for the prevention of functional decline: effect on higher-level physical function. Arch Phys Med Rehabil 2004;85(7):1043–9.
44. Gill TM, Baker DI, Gottschalk M, et al. A program to prevent functional decline in physically frail, elderly persons who live at home. N Engl J Med 2002;347(14): 1068–74.
45. Binder EF, Schechtman KB, Ehsani AA, et al. Effects of exercise training on frailty in community-dwelling older adults: results of a randomized, controlled trial. J Am Geriatr Soc 2002;50(12):1921–8.
46. Bandinelli S, Lauretani F, Boscherini V, et al. A randomized, controlled trial of disability prevention in frail older patients screened in primary care: the FRASI study. Design and baseline evaluation. Aging Clin Exp Res 2006;18(5):359–66.
47. Peterson MJ, Sloane R, Cohen HJ, et al. Effect of telephone exercise counseling on frailty in older veterans: project LIFE. Am J Mens Health 2007;1(4):326–34.
48. Fairhall N, Aggar C, Kurrle SE, et al. Frailty intervention trial (FIT). BMC Geriatr 2008;8:27.

49. Latham NK, Anderson CS, Lee A, et al. A randomized, controlled trial of quadriceps resistance exercise and vitamin D in frail older people: the Frailty Interventions Trial in Elderly Subjects (FITNESS). J Am Geriatr Soc 2003;51(3):291–9.
50. Schneider JK, Eveker A, Bronder DR, et al. Exercise training program for older adults. Incentives and disincentives for participation. J Gerontol Nurs 2003; 29(9):21–31.
51. Teri L, Gibbons LE, McCurry SM, et al. Exercise plus behavioral management in patients with Alzheimer disease: a randomized controlled trial. JAMA 2003; 290(15):2015–22.
52. Available at: www.health.gov/paguidelines/guidelines/default.aspx. Accessed February 1, 2010.

Index

Note: Page numbers of article titles are in **boldface** type.

A

Activities of daily living, regular physical activity and, 102–103
Aging, accumulation of deficits with, 17, 18
    and deficit accumulation, 21
    and frailty, biology of, **27–37**
    diminished ability to respond to stress in, 18
    hallmarks of, 39
    normal, 27–28
    onset of, and progression of, varying, 27
Anemia, and hemoglobin concentration, 67, 68
    IL-6 and, 71–72
    in frailty, **67–78**
    in older adults, consequences of, 68–69
        diagnosis of, clinical tests in, 70
        incidence of, 69
    interventions for consideration in, 73–74
    normocytic normochromic, 71
    of aging, population-based study groups and, 68
    of unexplained cause, 72–73
    peripheral white cells and, 72
    prevalence in older adults, 67–68
    treatment of, in elderly, 73
Angiotensin-converting enzyme, 53
Angiotensin-converting enzyme inhibitors, for treatment of osteoporosis, fracture risk,
    and bone marrow density, 59
    in prevention of myocardial infarction, 58
Angiotensin II, 53
    formation of, biochemical pathway of, 53, 54
Angiotensin receptors, changes with aging and/or frailty, 56, 57
Anti-inflammatory intervention, in frailty, 93–94
Apoptosis, and DNA damage, 28
    as controlled cellular demolition, 30
    initiation of, 29–30
Atherosclerosis, angiotensin II receptor blockers in prevention of, 58
Atrial fibrillation, angiotensin II receptor blockers in prevention of, 58

B

B-cell alteration, in frailty, 84
"Biologic age", frailty and, 22–23
Bone marrow density, fracture risk, osteoporosis, angiotensin-converting enzyme inhibitors
    for treatment of, 59

Clin Geriatr Med 27 (2011) 111–116
doi:10.1016/S0749-0690(10)00105-9
0749-0690/11/$ – see front matter © 2011 Elsevier Inc. All rights reserved.

geriatric.theclinics.com

Printed in the United States
By Bookmasters